Wigged Out!

Surviving Chemo and Other Intrusions

Cheryl Peyton

Copyright © 2020 by Cheryl Peyton

All rights reserved. No part of this book may be reproduced in any manner without the express written consent of the author, except in the case of brief excerpts in critical reviews.

This is a work of non-fiction. All dates and procedures correspond to a diary I kept on the course of my treatments throughout a year.

ISBN: 979-8671433715

This book was printed in the United States of America

Cover and illustrations by Cheryl Peyton

OTHER BOOKS BY CHERYL PEYTON

Six Minutes to Midnight

Walk on Through the Rain

Murder on Bedford Island

Murder on the Bermuda Queen

Murder in Margaritaville

Murder in Montmartre

Murder on the Rhine

Murder in Mobile

Conversations with Cody; A sassy Canine Speaks his Mind

Available in soft cover at www.amazon.com, www.authorsguildoftn.org and in select local stores.

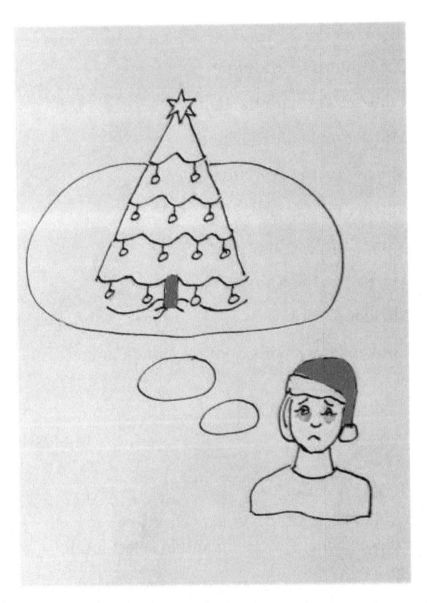

I'm wishing for any kind of Christmas

Chapter One

A Not-So-Merry Christmas

December 15, 2018

Ten days before Christmas in 2018 I discovered a lump in my right breast. That was *not* what I wanted for Christmas. I kept trying to tell myself that it was just a cyst that would disappear. However, it was still there the next day and the next, until I had to accept the possibility that the lump was a malignant tumor.

I wasn't just being dramatic. Seventeen years earlier, when I lived near Chicago, I had found a similar lump in my left breast that was cancerous. It was particularly upsetting at the time since only four months earlier I had barely survived a ruptured appendix and two years before that I had undergone surgery for rectal cancer.

I was starting to build a sizable portfolio of medical reports and evaluations that always described me in clinical terms such as: "The patient is a well-developed, well-nourished, white female in no acute distress." One report described me as a "58-year-old right-handed Glenview resident." *That's a demographic?*

When I discovered my lump in 2001, I was a patient of a gynecologist at Lake Forest Hospital in Illinois. Treatment was swift. An ultrasound confirmed the diagnosis on a Friday and I underwent a lumpectomy on the following Monday. The tumor was described as an "infiltrating ductal carcinoma, Grade III."

A few weeks later, after healing from surgery, I started on a three-month course of chemotherapy at Evanston hospital. A month after that I began daily radiation treatments at Glenbrook Hospital that lasted for four weeks. It was a rough seven months of enduring headaches, nausea, lethargy and other side effects. When I was released by my oncologist from needing further treatment, I still had low energy and was bald as a coot; but I was on the mend and grateful to be cancer-free.

* * *

In 2003 my husband Jim and I moved to a retirement community outside Knoxville, Tennessee. Our primary care physician at the time referred me to the Cancer Care of East Tennessee Clinic in the Tower at Parkwest Hospital for follow-up screenings. For over two years as a patient there my oncological exams, blood analyses, and mammograms were always negative.

* * *

Now, fourteen years later, and almost twenty years after my first breast cancer, I could be facing a recurrence of the disease. It was hard for me to believe I'd be going through the sickness and treatments all again.

It was a turbulent and confusing time in my personal life. While I was still living with Jim, my husband of many years, I had initiated a separation agreement. I had recently closed on the purchase of a house nearby, a neglected rental property that was in need of a total renovation. I had already contracted with a builder to do some remodeling, including redoing the master bath, installing vinyl flooring on the main level, and building a stacked-stone fireplace over the existing opening. I planned on doing all the cosmetic work myself. It was a daunting proposition to paint the entire interior and exterior trim of the three-bedroom house, but I had had years of experience working on other homes.

As I contemplated all that lay ahead, I called the Comprehensive Breast Center to advise them that I had found a lump and requested they move up my annual mammogram appointment that was scheduled for January 11. They told me that I would need a Diagnostic Mammogram that required a physician's referral. Okay. I called my primary doctor's office to request one, but was informed that she was off for the holidays and wouldn't be back until the second week in January.

"Couldn't she be contacted to just send a referral?" I protested. The response was not reassuring. They'd *attempt* to reach her, but they couldn't promise anything. Would I like to see another doctor for an examination when they could "fit me in?" No, thanks.

I decided I could wait a couple of days for my doctor to come through with a referral, although she was probably on some cruise and not concerned with patients back home who may have lumps in their breasts.

I spent the next few days working on the new house as a distraction. My husband helped me first pull up the carpeting and padding in the living area, which was a big help.

I couldn't do much more in that room until a painter spray-painted the vaulted knotty pine ceiling. I think originally it was supposed to look like a chalet in Switzerland, but by then it looked more like a bar in Sheboygan. The same kind of pine boards were on the downstairs office ceiling. Since the rooms were empty and undecorated, I thought it would be an easy job to spray the ceilings without even needing to put down drop cloths. Unfortunately, the contractor's painter had other jobs to finish before he could get to mine. It could be another week or two.

In the meantime, I called my doctor's office again, but they still hadn't received a referral. I decided the best way to ignore the orange ceilings and my possible breast cancer was to get back to work.

The project I started on was painting the oak-stained kitchen cabinets.

First, I took off all the hardware and set the twenty-nine doors and eight drawers against the living room walls in the same order they were in the kitchen.

Then, getting down on my hands and knees, I began painting with a small roller. After I finished a few doors, I realized the light grey wasn't covering well, and when it dried, the finish was chalky. After two coats it didn't look much better. I then made the fateful decision to go over everything with a clear satin polyurethane. As thinly as I applied it and with a good quality brush, the build-up in the corners and along the edges of the moldings turned orange. It seemed I couldn't get away from that color in this house. Now what?

I spent the next two days first sanding the varnish and then repainting with two coats on everything in a dark grey. The doors then looked pretty good. At least they weren't orange.

After that job, I carried a ladder upstairs to the master bedroom to begin scraping off the "popcorn" ceiling. Putting on goggles, a construction mask, and a headscarf, I started in the farthest corner of the room, knocking off the top layer with a steel scraper, using just enough pressure to remove it without gouging the plaster. It was grueling and messy work. As the crumbled plaster rained down on me, I had to stop every few minutes to clear the goggles and pull down the mask to breathe. Progress was slow.

After an hour or so, I heard someone knocking on the front door. Who could that be? I wasn't expecting anyone.

Getting off the ladder, I removed my mask and goggles and shook out the scarf and headed downstairs. Cautiously opening the door, I was amazed to see a man standing there who was obviously a painter. Over his shoulder I could read his company name on the side of the panel truck in the driveway.

I excitedly invited him in and pointed out the ceiling above us, then walked him down the hallway to show him the other one.

Looking around, he nodded. "Easy job."

Good to his word, within a couple of hours, he had sprayed both ceilings a creamy white. They looked so much better that I felt optimistic about everything.

The next day, I was inspired to write a parody of the poem, "The Night Before Christmas," to keep up my good spirits:

The Week Before Christmas

'Twas the week before Christmas, but in my new house
There weren't any candles or evergreen boughs.
No stockings were hung by the chimney with care;
There was no sign that St. Nicholas would ever be there.

Nor could I nestle all snug in my bed.
As I hadn't moved in yet; only worked there, instead.

So, I in my kerchief, goggles, and mask
Started scraping a ceiling to check off one task -
When out on the driveway there arose such a clatter,
I sprang from my perch to see what was the matter.

Away to the window I flew like a flash --
Peered through a pane to see what caused the crash.
When what to my wondering eyes did appear,
But a professional painter with all of his gear.

In his right hand he carried a power paint sprayer.
He would cover my orange ceiling, an answer to prayer.
More rapid than eagles through the front door he came,
Put down his equipment; said Kris was his name.

He was dressed all in white from his head to his shoes
(Except for dried paint drops in various hues).
The bundle of tools he had flung over his back
Made him look like a peddler toting his pack.

He spoke very little but went straight to his work
Filling his sprayer, he turned with a jerk
And, laying his finger aside of his nose,
Gave me a nod and up the ladder he rose.

He pressed on his nozzle to release a fine flow
That blanketed the ceiling like new fallen snow.
The orangey pine boards were now covered in white
Which opened the space and gave it more light.
When he finished, he smiled with a twinkle in his eye;

Then drove off so quickly, it was like he could fly.

I sat in a daze long after he left.
Kris had made me believe I'd have a nice Christmas yet!

* * *

A few days later, Jim and I celebrated Christmas, having dinner at one of the few restaurants in the area that was open on the holiday. He asked me if I was still worried about having cancer since I seemed to be in such a good mood of late. I said I had decided to put it out of my mind, knowing that I had an appointment for a mammogram on January 11. I didn't admit I hadn't been successful at this, but I think he knew. We talked about other things and had a good time.

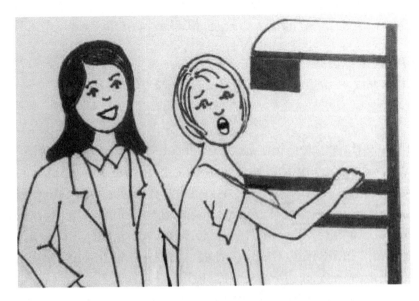

"I know it's a little uncomfortable, Mrs. Peyton, but you just need to hold your breath and not move for a few minutes."

Chapter Two

The Diagnosis

January 17, 2019

Right after New Year's three Hispanic men appeared at my door with boxes of stones. The youngest man explained his father was there to build my new fireplace and he and the other man were helpers.

I was very glad to see them as I couldn't paint the living room and the other adjoining walls until the floor-to-ceiling fireplace was in place.

I noticed that the stones were divided into the three boxes according to their light, medium, and dark earth tones. I told the young man that I hoped the lighter stones would be used as much as possible rather than the dark ones. He just nodded in a non-committal way.

I thought I'd try out my college Spanish with the stonemason to be sure he understood, except that I couldn't remember the Spanish words for 'stones,' or 'rocks,' or even, 'lighter.' I was left with pointing and saying "no mucho negro o café (not much of the black or brown). Then, holding up a light stone, I announced, "Me gusta esto." (I like this.)

I'm sure he thought I was a nut case, but he was nice enough to try to reassure me that he understood. He picked up one of the light-colored stones and said, "Te gusta piedra de colores mas claro," which I then figured out meant, "You like lighter stones like this."

"Sí, sí," I said, lamely.

The fireplace turned out great. The stonemason was a true artisan and he used all the light stones he had. He also managed somehow to stack stones of different sizes and shapes and kept straight horizontal lines.

Soon afterwards, I painted the living room, hallways, and staircases. When I was finished, I had only three days to wait until my mammogram appointment. The Comprehensive Breast Center assured me that they would follow up with a diagnostic mammogram if they saw "anything suspicious" in the regular one.

I showed up early for my January 11 appointment, eager to have the scan done, although I felt it would be just a preliminary picture. The technician who took the X-rays didn't comment on the mass in my left breast, but the next day the Center called me to schedule a diagnostic mammogram for the following week. I finally had a date and time to find out definitively if I had cancer or not.

* * *

On January 17, I walked into the Center with trepidation. This was it. I was prepared for the worst; determined not to fall apart. There was always a chance that the mass was some other kind of abnormality.

After checking in with the office staff to verify my personal information like name, address, and insurance company, a nurse came out to take me back to a room. She paused at the doorway to ask me my birthdate. (Personnel in a medical setting always ask you for your birthdate to verify you are who you say you are. I mean, I could have been an imposter trying to get a mammogram meant for someone else.)

She then led me down a hallway and into an examining room where she sat at a computer to record my answers regarding medical history. After she took my temperature and blood pressure, she handed me a seersucker gown to change into, telling me that it should "open in front." *Really?*

She returned a few minutes later to take me to the same X-ray room where I had the regular mammogram the week before. The difference with the diagnostic, I soon discovered, was that they took more images and the steel plates were pressed even more tightly together. It was all I could do not to cry out.

After that was over and I caught my breath, I followed the nurse into another examining room where a technologist introduced herself and asked me for my birthdate. I wanted to say it was the same as it was a half hour earlier, but refrained.

She instructed me to lie down on the examining table and then opened my gown on my right side. (I would become used to having my breast exposed to sundry medical personnel over the coming months.)

She then explained that the radiologist would first do an ultrasound to find the "exact location" of the mass and then take a sample for the biopsy. I was thinking that I could just point to the spot, but . . . whatever.

The doctor came in and went over the two procedures with me. "This won't be too bad," he assured me. *"Not too bad"* sounded pretty bad to me.

He sat down facing a screen next to the machine, then picked up the transducer probe and slathered gel on it. He commenced rolling the cold, hard disk over the tender area around the mass, which was *very* uncomfortable, contrary to what he had said. After a few minutes, I thought he should be done, but he kept going. Finally, he made some marks on my chest and put down the probe.

The nurse wiped off the gel with paper toweling, then swabbed me with a cotton ball soaked in sterilizing solution and applied what she said was a topical anesthesia.

The doctor explained he would be using a fine needle to draw out a small sample, that the needle was even finer than the kind used for drawing blood. I thought, that may be true, but they don't draw blood from your breast.

I looked away as he inserted the needle at the location he had marked. I don't care how fine that needle was, it hurt like the dickens. Fortunately, it didn't take long, but I took a deep breath in relief when he extracted it.

Patting my shoulder, he told me I did very well. *At least I hadn't jumped off the table.* As the nurse cleaned up the room, the doctor explained that he would be reviewing my X-rays and a pathologist would examine the breast tissue sample under a microscope to determine its molecular composition. I should expect a phone call in the next day or two.

I tried to read something in the doctor's face, but he wasn't giving anything away.

* * *

Two days later I was at the house scraping ceilings again while the construction crew was tearing out the master bath. Between the sledge hammering, the country music playing at full volume, and the plaster dust in the air, it was total chaos.

In the afternoon, I heard my cell phone ringtone. The caller ID read "Covenant Health." I knew it was the Comprehensive Breast Center calling and immediately picked up and said, "Hello." No response. I had noticed that cell phone service wasn't good inside the house, so I raced to the front door and ran out into the cold air.

"HELLO? CAN YOU HEAR ME NOW?" I yelled.

"Yes," I heard a woman say at a normal level. "Is this Cheryl?"

"Yes, this is she," I responded, sheepishly.

The caller identified herself as the supervising nurse at the clinic. She asked if this was a good time to talk or I could call her back when it was.

I explained that I was outside on my cell phone that didn't have a strong signal, but I was fine to talk.

She apologized for keeping me out in the cold, then paused. "Uh, the pathologist has examined the biopsy of the tissue from your right breast."

"Yes?" I said to encourage her to go on.

"I'm sorry to tell you," she continued, "but your biopsy revealed that the mass is cancerous."

My eyes filled with tears. "Yes . . . I thought so."

She went on to explain that the clinic had already made an appointment for me to meet with Dr. William Gibson at Parkwest the following Monday. She assured me that he was their best surgeon.

I said I appreciated that and thanked her for calling and for making the appointment.

I disconnected and went back into the house, ready to take up my scraper again. The work would keep my mind occupied. Besides, I had only three days before I'd see Dr. Gibson and start on the process of having the tumor removed and receiving treatments.

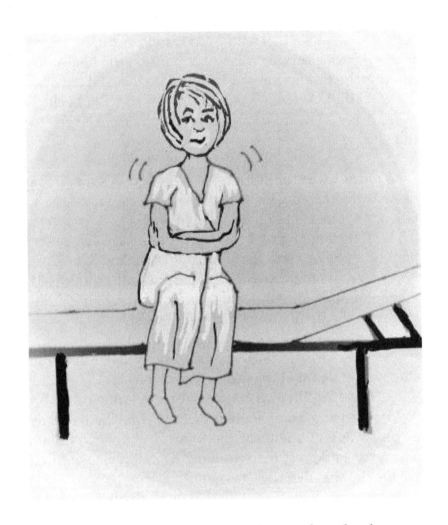

I don't know if I'm nervous about what the doctor will say or it's just so darn cold in here.

Chapter Three

I'm Not a Patient Patient

January 24, 2019

At the appointed time on the following Monday, Jim and I arrived at the offices of Dr. Gibson's surgical group and checked in. After several minutes, a nurse came out to take us back to an examining room. Once inside, I handed Jim my coat and purse and sat in the chair next to the computer where the nurse was typing. She asked me a few preliminary questions and then wrapped a blood pressure cuff around my arm. "Excellent blood pressure," she commented. I smiled as I'm usually asked if it is normally *so low*.

Standing up, she reached for a clean, folded hospital gown and handed it to me. "You just need to undress to the waist. Put this on—with the front open. Dr. Gibson will be in shortly to talk to you."

I thanked her and after she left, I did as she said and sat on the padded table to wait, shivering in the flimsy wrap since the room was about 60 degrees. Jim and I looked at our watches.

Before long, there was a knock on the door and Dr. Gibson came in, followed by the nurse. I was pleased to see that he was a man in his mid-40's, the age group I've always considered the most desirable for doctors; knowing they've had 15-20 years in practice, and assuming that they're up to date on the latest research.

After introductions, Dr. Gibson pursed his lips as he glanced at the open folder he was holding. "I've been going over your file. I see you were treated for cancer in your left breast back in 2001, but I don't have the medical records. Can you tell me what all you had done at that time?" He leaned back against the wall of cabinets, looking relaxed. A good sign, I thought.

I told him all that was done in Illinois at Lake Forest Hospital, Evanston, and Glenbrook. It sounded like I had been hospital-shopping, but he didn't react.

"Were any lymph glands removed in the surgery?" he asked.

I told him that the sentinel node and one other node in the left armpit had been removed to biopsy while I was being operated on. Since the nodes were cancer-free, no other nodes were removed."

He nodded and smiled in approval. "Good. I'll be doing the same. Did the surgeon make any cosmetic repairs with the lumpectomy?"

"I don't think so," I answered, uncertainly.

"Well, let's have a look," he said. The nurse came around and eased me back on the table that was elevated slightly at the head.

Dr. Gibson gently parted my gown. Pursing his lips, he inspected the scar and depression in my left breast, then shook his head. "Oh, this doesn't look good."

"Thanks," I said.

He chuckled. "Sorry. I meant there hasn't been any re-contouring of the breast. When I operate, I'll go in through the areola to avoid making an incision in the outside of the breast itself."

My eyes widened in surprise.

He held up a hand. "That way you won't have a scar like you have on the left side. Then I'll move some breast tissue to fill in the space where the tumor was. You won't see any difference in the size and shape you have now. I think you'll be pleased with the result."

I twisted my mouth, considering. "I guess the lumpectomy technique has advanced over the years since I had mine done."

Dr. Gibson's eyebrows rose slightly. "I was doing it the same way in 2001 that I do now," he answered.

Pulling a stethoscope out of his pocket, he listened to my heart and lungs. Satisfied, he closed my gown and stepped over to the counter while I sat up and scooted to the end of the table.

He picked up his folder again and flipped through a couple pages until he stopped to look at one. Laying down the folder, he stroked his chin. "I, uh, looked carefully at your ultrasound pictures and read through the pathology report." He paused. "I have to tell you...I don't like the look of that cancer."

I blinked, not sure what he meant.

"It's a Grade III. That's the most aggressive type of cancer cell when examined under a microscope. You may be more familiar with the stages of cancer. They relate to the tumor's size and its degree of spread to surrounding tissue." Grades refer to how abnormal the cells are in terms of how likely they can spread."

I felt my face flush. I had the most abnormal kind of cancer cells?

The doctor continued. "We can't be sure without doing more scans, but my fear is that there may well be some cancerous cells that have traveled elsewhere in your body. For that reason, I want you to go through chemotherapy before I operate."

My mouth dropped open. I was sure that I would be undergoing surgery as soon as possible as I had years before.

He looked me in the eye. "I'm sure this is the best way to go. If there are stray cancer cells, they'll be eradicated with the chemo. Also, I expect that the tumor will be shrunk down, maybe to nothing, after the chemo."

I looked at Jim. He half-shrugged. It sounded reasonable to him.

I nodded, then dropped my head. It had been a whole month since I first felt the lump and fixated on having it taken out. Now surgery would be put off for months.

Dr. Gibson wasn't through with the bad news. "You're going to need an MRI before starting chemo so we can get a complete picture of the soft tissues in your chest and abdomen to see if there are any hot spots."

I bit my lip.

"We can get that scheduled soon." he added.

"I felt the tumor before Christmas," I said, my voice wavering. "I'm worried that it's been growing since then."

Dr. Gibson shook his head. "They don't grow that fast. That tumor has probably been there for several months — up to a year."

I wasn't sure if that was good news or bad.

He raised an index finger. "One more thing. I'll need to insert a port before you get chemotherapy. That way, they won't have to stick you each time. It's much easier on the patient. Did you have a port when you got chemo years ago?"

I shook my head. "No."

"Well, that's another advance, then. Okay, I'll leave you to get dressed. When you're ready, step across the hall to the scheduling desk and they'll set you up at Parkwest for an MRI on the first available date and find a date for me to insert the port."

A took a breath. "Okay. Good."

He patted my shoulder. "Don't worry. We're going to take good care of you and get rid of that tumor as soon as we can. I know it takes more time than you'd like, but we're on top of things now."

I managed a smile. "Thanks, Dr. Gibson."

After he left, I dressed and Jim and I walked out into the hallway to see that the scheduling department was only a few feet away.

The intake worker said she had all my information and she'd just be a minute making a couple calls. When she hung up on the second one, she handed me two appointment cards: one for an MRI at Parkwest on January 25, and a card for the port insertion on February 5.

It'll all work out, I told myself. I just need to have a little more patience.

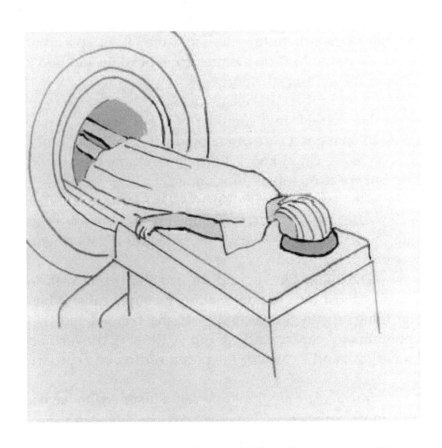

Wouldn't it be funny if there's no one still out there to get me out of this contraption?

Chapter Four

Testing my Patience

January 25, 2019

Around mid-morning on the 25th, I drove up to the main entrance of Parkwest hospital and pulled into the patient's valet lane. A young man hustled over, opened my door and greeted me. As I got out of the car, he politely asked for my last name and wrote it on the top of a ticket, then handed me the lower half. As I took it and started to walk away, he said, "Have a wonderful day." *I'm going into the hospital. How wonderful can it be?*

Once inside, I made my way across the busy lobby to the patient registration desk where I checked in. I was handed a pager and told to have a seat. Squeezing between two others in the crowded waiting room, I settled back with my beeper in hand. To pass the time I looked around at the other patients, idly wondering why they were there and was startled when my pager lit up and buzzed after only a few minutes. An intake worker called my name and I followed her down a hallway past several offices and then into one.

As I sat across the desk from her, she asked for my birthdate and other identifying information that she checked on her screen. Satisfied she had all that she needed, she printed a queue of papers and a page full of stickers while she rattled off what I would be signing where she had hi-lighted.

After slapping the stickers on the papers, she passed the sheets to me one at a time, giving me only enough time to scrawl my name on each. From what I could gather glancing through them, they were mostly concerned with indemnifying the hospital, its physicians, and all other personnel for whatever services and treatment they deemed necessary for my care. The last questions didn't inspire confidence either: "Do you have a living will?" and, "Who should we call in the event of an emergency?" Finally, I signed that I agreed to be personally responsible for whatever charges there would be.

The registrar turned to scan down a screen on her computer. "I see your copay for today is $220," she chirped. "Will that be a charge?"

Yikes. I hadn't expected to pay that much. After she swiped my card, she snapped a plastic ID bracelet on me and thanked me for choosing Parkwest. "Do you need me to take you over to the outpatient waiting room?" she asked. I told her thanks, but I knew the way.

Back out in the atrium, I walked past the curved staircase that goes down to the cafeteria, and continued on to the glass-walled waiting room where I checked in at the desk. The receptionist gave me a pager and asked me to have a seat, saying it shouldn't be long. There were at least a dozen other people there for a variety of scans and radioactive imaging.

While I waited, I looked at the television that was tuned in to HGTV, like all sets at Parkwest, and watched a home remodeling show for a few minutes before a male technician came out and called my name.

We chatted about the weather as he took me down three hallways to a room with lockers that he instructed me to use for my clothes after changing into the short-sleeved gown he handed me.

Minutes later he returned and tapped on the door. I went with him around a corner to a closed door at the end of a short hallway. The low-lit room inside was dominated by a hulking space-age tubular machine that had one round opening. A padded table sat just outside the machine.

The room was cold enough to hang meat. I rubbed my arms and blew out my breath expecting to see it. The technician apologized for the cool temperature, explaining that it was necessary for the machine to function properly. He went on to explain that the imaging was done by a magnetic field of radio waves.

He then handed me a pair of earphones he said would help block out the tapping, thumping, and other noises the magnet produced. "Sorry we don't have music," he said. I shrugged to indicate I didn't mind.

He said that the exam should take only about half an hour. *Only? That's a long time to be stuck in that tube.*

As requested, I lay face down on the table. The cushion was covered in stiff vinyl that didn't give. I squirmed around to try to get comfortable, but I felt little support where I needed it. The only accommodation to my anatomy appeared to be the opening in the table for my chest.

The technician then had me put my face down on a hard, circular form. I tried to lift my head a little to take some of my weight off my forehead, but I soon realized I couldn't do that for long. My next maneuver was to lift my body with my hands that were down by my sides. I felt like a seal holding up his weight on his flippers. I didn't remember massage therapists' tables being this uncomfortable.

Once I had achieved enough rigidity to hold my body up a little, I was pleasantly surprised when the technician brought a warmed blanket that he draped over me. I suddenly felt much better.

He then went over to the wall and flipped the switch to darken the room and called out, "Ready? Here we go."

The table I was on moved into the tube as the machine started a low whirring. Despite the earphones I realized I still could hear like a Doberman Pinscher.

For the next half an hour my ears were assaulted with knocks, buzzing, and whining like you'd hear in a horror movie.

During the time I was being moved in and out of the tube, I continued to lift myself with my hands and my neck alternately, being careful to hold still when I heard noises from the machine so that the pictures wouldn't be blurry and I'd have to do this again.

Finally, it was quiet. The technician came over to check on me and pulled me to a sitting position. He asked if I thought I could stand. Good question. I replied that I thought I could and he helped me off the table.

As we walked out of the room, I was quite wobbly, so he held my right elbow. When we got back to the changing room, he suggested I sit for a while and take my time getting dressed to make sure I was stable enough to drive home.

I followed his advice. After maybe ten minutes, I felt my plugged ears clear up enough to regain my balance. After dressing, I splashed cold water on my face and felt ready to go.

On my way out of the hospital through the atrium, I looked around for a friend I knew was having a test that day, but I didn't see her.

Outside, at the valet station, I ran into another friend who was waiting for her daughter to pick her up. Dianna told me she had just gotten steroid shots in the back of her neck to relieve pain, but the shots themselves were so painful she wasn't sure it was worth it.

As I drove off, I thought that it's a sad day when you can see more friends at the hospital than you'll run into at the grocery store. At least the three of us were all out-patients. Something to be thankful for.

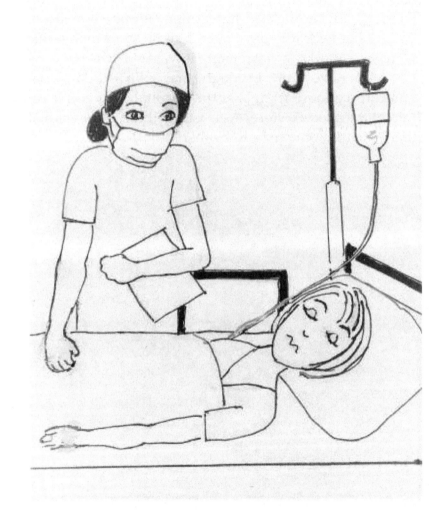

"You haven't gotten the anesthetic yet, Mrs. Peyton. This is just saline to hydrate you."

Chapter Five

My First Surgery

February 5, 2019

Jim and I had to set our GPS to find the clinic where I'd have my port inserted. We knew it was located off Papermill Road, but wasn't visible from the street. The modest one-story building sat hidden between two commercial businesses. As we stepped out of the car after the voice on the GPS said we had arrived, the only indication it was a bustling medical operation was a small sign on the door that read, "Premier Surgical Associates."

Passing through the glass doors, we checked in with the receptionist behind the high counter and were asked to take a seat in the small waiting area, joining a few other patients.

It wasn't long before a nurse came out for us. We followed her down a hallway until she ushered us into a windowless room that was sparsely furnished with two straight-backed chairs, a computer, and a hospital bed. I noticed how chilly the room was.

The nurse invited us to sit while she took my temperature and blood pressure. "Are your numbers always that low?" she asked, referring to my 97 over 56 reading.

"That's typical for me," I assured her.

She nodded. "Have you had anything to eat or drink since midnight?"

"No, not since maybe eight o'clock," I replied.

She held out a hospital gown. "Okay, good. I'm going to step outside for you to change into this. Take everything off except your panties. Then, you can get into the bed and I'll be back to get your IV going."

I did as she asked, but once in bed, I was shivering having only a sheet to pull over me.

Thankfully, the nurse soon came back carrying two blankets that had been warmed, draping one over me and giving Jim the other.

Feeling more comfortable, I relaxed and turned my left arm for the nurse to swab and stick me with a needle. She then connected it to an IV tube that went up to the plastic bag overhead. I thought of the irony of getting an IV to prepare me for a port to avoid IVs.

"This is just saline," she said as I closed my eyes, already drifting off by the suggestion of being put to sleep. "The anesthesiologist will be in soon and then Dr. Gibson will come to talk to you."

"Uh, huh," I murmured, pulling the blanket up to my chin.

I opened my eyes when the anesthesiologist came in to ask questions about whether I had any allergies to medications and how I did previously with being anesthetized.

I advised him that I had been told I slept a little longer in the recovery room, but within a normal range.

He nodded. "I think you'll do fine. You'll be in more of a twilight state than completely under."

Dr. Gibson came in later and went over the procedure. "This will probably take less than an hour. As you recall, I'm going to implant a small reservoir under your skin and insert the attached tube into a vein. During your treatment, they'll access the port for all infusions and for blood drawings. You can expect the area will be sore for about a week and you'll need to keep the bandaging dry until it heals; so take baths or cover it when you shower. Do you have any questions?"

I shook my head.

"Okay, if you're ready, I am. Let's get going."

I became dimly aware that my bed was being moved and I saw Jim wave at me as I closed my eyes again and waited for the darkness to envelop me.

* * *

I awoke to find myself fully dressed in bed in a darkened room with other patients in beds nearby — the recovery unit. I tried to make sense of how I had my clothes back on. Jim sat in a chair nearby so I asked him.

"The nurses dressed you. I was outside so I don't know how they managed. You must have helped them a little. You don't remember?"

"No, I don't remember anything about it. Well, it's a good thing you're driving. I might not remember the way home."

* * *

As Dr. Gibson had said, the area around the port was sore for the next week. I was careful to sleep on my left side and not move my right shoulder during the day. For showering, I taped a plastic bag over the bandaging. After several days, I barely noticed the nickel-sized bump just under my collarbone. I was happy to be ready to receive chemotherapy and hoped it would be soon.

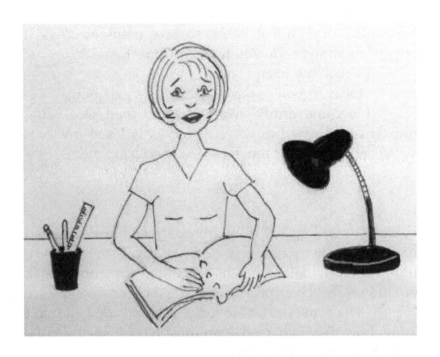

"I think I've read enough about nausea, hair loss, fatigue, loss of appetite, bone pain, and skin rashes. Egads."

Chapter Six

Tennessee Cancer Specialists

February 12, 2019

The day finally arrived when I had an appointment at Tennessee Cancer Specialists, the chemotherapy clinic affiliated with Parkwest hospital.

A little before 1:30 p.m. Jim pulled into the parking lot of the contemporary grey and white building on Sherrill Boulevard, less than a mile away from the hospital.

Walking inside, we found ourselves in a circular, sunshine filled atrium. I gave my name to the receptionist behind the curved desk who advised that we would be meeting with a nurse and gestured to her right where we would find a small waiting room.

"I'll let Chrissy know you're here," she said as we started in the direction she indicated.

We hadn't waited long when a young, dark-haired woman came out and called my name. She introduced herself and asked us to follow her back to her office. Once we were seated across the desk from her, she explained that she was my Nurse Navigator who would coordinate my care during my time there as a patient. She said that it would be her job to educate me about my disease and treatment, to make any outside appointments, help me manage side effects, and, of course, provide emotional support. It sounded like a tall order.

She handed me a loose-leaf notebook that was titled "Patient Resource Guide." We spent the rest of the hour going through the twelve tabbed sections to acquaint me with the contents and how to best use the material. Besides contact information and lined pages for me to write in appointments and medications, there were chapters titled, "Drug Information," "Side Effects and Symptoms Management," "Cancer Terms," and finally, "Survivorship Plans." I noticed the longest chapters were on side effects and how to manage the symptoms.

When she finished with her descriptions of each chapter, she asked if I had any questions. I had a lot of questions, but the first one was, "When will I start my chemotherapy sessions?"

Chrissy looked down at her desk and shuffled a couple of papers before picking one up. "It says here you have an appointment with your oncology physician, Dr. Feng (pronounced Fung), this next Friday on the 15th."

I brightened and looked over at Jim.

Chrissy twisted her mouth. "Uh, I'm not sure if he'll start you on chemo then, but you'll have your blood drawn and he'll examine you and go over your medical history." She glanced down at her paper again. "I see he's ordered four to six 21-day cycles of Taxotere, Cytoxan and Neulasta, for three to four months."

It took me a minute to do the math, but it sounded like the treatments would take me from February into the summer. I swallowed hard.

Before we left, Chrissy had me sign a form titled "Consent to Receive Chemotherapy at Tennessee Cancer Specialists." Blank spaces had been filled in with my chemotherapy drugs and the schedule that had been ordered by Dr. Feng. The form's pre-printed language contained paragraphs that began with "I understand"

and went on to include all the possible effects and outcomes of cancer treatment. The side effects included the common ones, like hair loss, vomiting, and anemia; more serious ones, like abdominal cramps, muscle aches and bone pain; and the most serious ones, like heart failure, lung toxicity, secondary cancers, and even death. Egads. This is the treatment I'm looking forward to?

On the ride home I was excited to talk over all we had been told, noting what was the same and what was different from my breast cancer treatment years earlier.

We would be back to the clinic in another three days when I would hopefully start my treatment.

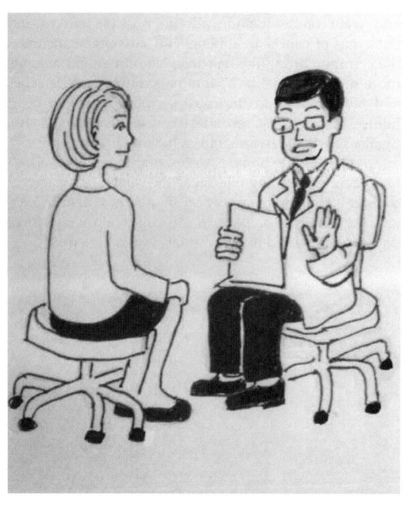

"We can't have too many pictures of your tumor, Mrs. Peyton."

Chapter Seven

My First Doctor's Appointment

February 15, 2019

When we returned to the clinic three days later it already felt routine, although this time the receptionist sent us to the large waiting area next to the Infusion room.

When I was called, I followed the nurse inside to have my blood drawn. I noticed that about half the recliners in the five rows were occupied. All the patients appeared to be relaxed; most were leaning back with their feet up, many were nestled under blankets, and some were sleeping.

One side of the room featured a glass wall that looked out to a courtyard planted with trees and bushes. If it weren't for the IV bags and tubes attached to the patients, you could have thought it was just another lounge area.

My nurse, Leslie, asked me to select any chair I liked. I picked the closest one and sat down. As she stood next to me, I pulled the collar of my shirt away from my neck to give her access to my new port.

"Oh, I can get to it easily," she said. "Is this your first time here?"

I told her it was the first time to see Dr. Feng, but my husband and I had met with my Nurse Navigator earlier in the week.

"You'll like Dr. Feng," she said. "He very kind and is a wonderful doctor."

I smiled and nodded. She then swabbed the area over my port and asked, "Did you put on some of the numbing cream at home?"

I answered that I had. She said if I ever forgot, not to worry, that it was just a little prick.

I didn't feel a thing as she stuck my port and drew out a couple of vials of blood. When she was finished, she directed me to go back through the reception area, and into the waiting room behind it where I'd be called in to see Dr. Feng.

Jim and I waited there several minutes before a nurse came out to call my name. She first weighed me and took my temperature before showing us back to an examining room. Another nurse came in to take my blood pressure and confirm information on my profile.

As she was leaving, she handed me a hospital gown to change into. "Down to the waist only. I'll be back with Dr. Feng shortly."

After a few minutes, there was a tap on the door and a slightly-built Asian man burst in, pumped my hand and then Jim's, as he introduced himself and said it was good to meet us. I noticed his accent made him a little hard to understand.

Dr. Feng's nurse followed him in and closed the door behind her. The doctor then perched on the edge of a stool across from me. He told me he had gone over my records and was familiar with my case. Holding up a page of columns with figures, he smiled. "Your blood work is good. All normal."

His face turned serious as he told me he wasn't satisfied with my MRI. Although it was good imagery of the tumor, it didn't give him information about the cancer cells. He wanted me to have a complete PET/CT scan that would take pictures of my skull down to mid-thigh. This, he said, would be definitive of the kind of cancer and how involved it was in my other systems.

Of course, I couldn't argue about needing the specialized test, but I was disappointed that there would be another delay in treating the tumor.

Dr. Feng instructed me to get up on the table where he listened to my heart and lungs and then examined my right breast, palpating it to feel the tumor.

As he picked up his papers to leave, he told me that the check-out people would have made the appointment for my PET/CT scan. As he opened the door, he waved and grinned. "See you soon," he said.

Out in the atrium area I gave my name to one of the women at the check-out counter. She pulled up my scheduled appointments, printed the page, and handed it to me. I saw that I had an appointment for a scan at the East Tennessee Diagnostic Center the following Monday, February 18, although it was pending authorization from Humana. I also had an appointment for chemotherapy at the clinic the next Friday, February 22nd.

One more week before treatment. I was getting close.

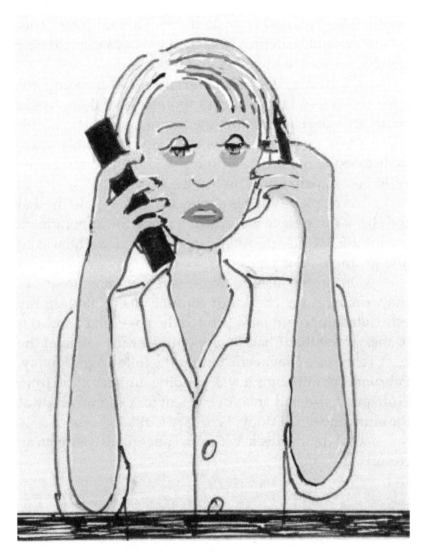

"Yes, I'll hold . . .maybe I'll get something to eat."

Chapter Eight

Is it a Scan or a Scam?

February 16-20, 2019

The following day when I hadn't heard from the cancer clinic or the East Tennessee Diagnostic Center, I called Chrissy, my Nurse Navigator, to see if she had received word that the PET/CT scans had been authorized by Humana. She said she hadn't heard anything and I should call the other clinic and Humana. I felt myself frown. I thought that was *her* job.

Since I was the one who needed to find out, I called the Diagnostic Center. They said they were waiting to hear from Humana.

I then called Humana and was transferred around, starting with Customer Service. They told me they didn't have any paperwork on the matter, and transferred me to the Intake Department. Intake advised me they had received the request and had passed it along to Authorizations. I was given my case number for reference.

I called the Authorizations' number and was connected with Stephanie, one of the agents. I gave her my case number. She left to check on it and came back on the line. Yes, they had the request, but the Review Board hadn't yet made a decision. She explained that it's unusual to receive a request for two scans together that included the skull down to mid-thigh. I couldn't argue with her. I did ask if she had some idea on how long it would take the Board to decide. I was scheduled to have my scans on Monday, two days from then. Not surprisingly, she couldn't guess how long the Board would need to review my medical file and decide whether to authorize payment, but they would notify Dr. Feng as soon as they had reached a decision.

I waited until the end of the day, Saturday, and then called Authorizations again. They hadn't yet made a decision on my case.

* * *

There didn't seem any point in trying to reach people on Sunday. The first thing Monday morning I called Humana's Authorizations department. This time they had an answer. The request for my two scans had been denied; they would pay for a CT scan of my abdomen and pelvis.

Would this be enough to satisfy Dr. Feng? Would it be sufficient to determine the extent of my cancer?

I called Tennessee Cancer Specialists and, following procedure, asked to speak to Chrissy. When she came on the line, I briefly relayed what I had learned from my phone calls with Humana, ending with the report of the Board's denial to authorize the two scans.

Chrissy told me that she thought the CT scan alone would be adequate, but would check with Dr. Feng and get back to me. She called me back in the afternoon to tell me that Dr. Feng was okay with a CT scan. What about my appointment at the Diagnostic Center? Chrissy said that Parkwest could do the CT and I should call them for an appointment. I didn't argue, but I again thought it was *her* job.

I called the radiation department at Parkwest to schedule a CT scan, telling them that I had my first appointment for chemo that Friday, February 22nd.

I was told they could work me in on Wednesday, February 20 at 5:00 p.m.

* * *

I arrived early for my appointment at Parkwest, although it was so late in the day there were only a few people around. I was the last appointment in the radiation department.

After a brief interview with the technician regarding my medical history, I changed into a gown and came out into a small waiting area where I was given a 16-ounce bottle of water to drink. When I managed to get that down, I was escorted to a darkened room that housed a donut-shaped machine.

When I lay down on the cot by the machine's opening, the technician stuck my wrist with a needle to connect me to an IV. He then left to operate the machine from an adjacent room. I was then shuttled in and out of the opening a few times while I held deep breaths and exhaled as directed by a recorded male voice.

After a few minutes I was told I would feel a warming sensation from the contrast material. A surge of heat spread up from my crotch. It felt odd, but not unpleasant.

After a few minutes, I was told it was over and I had done very well. I was happy I had made it over the last hurdle before starting chemotherapy in two days; it was now more than two months since I first felt the tumor.

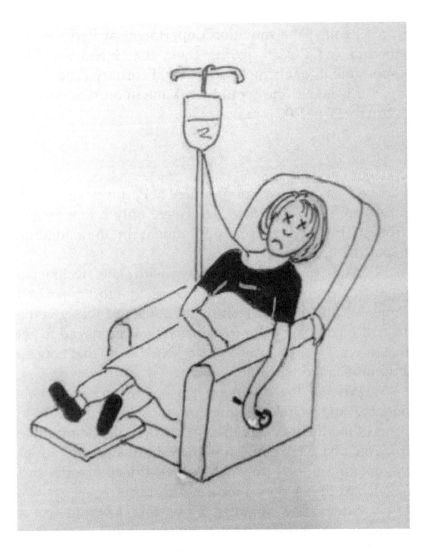

This just doesn't feel right.

Chapter Nine

My First Drugging

February 22, 2019

Jim turned into the parking lot of the Tennessee Cancer Specialists at 8:00 a.m. sharp. It was a cool, sunny day. Getting out of the car, I nearly sprinted toward the entrance, excited to receive my first chemotherapy after weeks of delays for tests and insurance approvals.

After checking in with the receptionist, we were directed to the seating area behind her to wait for my blood to be drawn and to see Dr. Feng.

As we sat, Jim mentioned that he needed to take the car in for an oil change and tire rotation. I suggested that he leave then and take care of it while I was being infused. He'd have time as the chemotherapy would take a couple of hours. He was reluctant, saying he didn't feel right leaving me for my first session; but neither did he want me to wait if he stopped on the way home. I assured him he didn't need to stay with me, that I would be well taken care of by the nurses. Besides, I had a book to read, or I could just rest. I had remembered to bring an afghan so I would be warm and comfortable in one of the reclining chairs.

We were still debating when a nurse called my name and I went into the lab with her to have my blood drawn through my port. I had applied the numbing cream so I didn't even feel the little prick. She filled a couple of vials and released me back to the waiting area.

In a few minutes, we were led back to an examining room to wait to see Dr. Feng who soon swept in carrying a sheaf of papers. "I have your CT scan results," he announced.

I held my breath. "And...?"

"There weren't any surprises," he said, looking down to read. "Soft tissues of the neck are normal, thyroid gland normal, some degenerative arthritis along your spine." He looked over at me. I nodded that I understood. "Most important," he went on, "no evidence of metastatic disease."

I smiled at hearing the best result I could hope for.

Dr Feng tapped on another paper. "Your blood work good, too, so you ready to have chemo today. I'll come back later to see how you're doing."

He opened the door for us to go back to sit by the Infusion Room. After a few minutes, a nurse came out to get me and we followed her back. I picked the recliner nearest the nurses' station. As I settled in, I told Jim he should leave and take care of the car. He gave a little nod.

"Okay. Call me if you need anything," he said before he walked away.

The nurse accessed my port with a needle and connected a tube that went up to the bag of steroids. She started the drip and the bag emptied in about twenty minutes. She came back when the beeper sounded and asked how I felt. I said I was fine.

She changed bags. "I'm going to start the Taxodere," she said. "Since this is your first time, I'll stay close and keep an eye on you. Let me know *immediately* if you feel *any different*. If you feel heat, or feel faint — anything different."

The Taxodere drip started. The nurse checked the flow before she walked away. I sat up straighter in my chair to read my book, pulling the afghan around me. I had read only one paragraph when my face felt flushed and I had to gasp for air. I opened my mouth to call out but I didn't have enough breath or voice. I could only wave my arms clumsily to get attention.

Within seconds there were nurses coming at me from all directions. One nurse covered my mouth and nose with an oxygen mask while another one yanked out my IV tube and attached another one in my port. A third nurse wrapped a blood pressure cuff around my arm.

Dr. Feng suddenly appeared and asked me how I felt. I had enough breath by then to tell him I was doing better. At least I wasn't about to pass out.

He patted my shoulder. "You be okay now," he said. I still felt overheated and light-headed. I pushed the afghan off my lap, leaned back and took some deep breaths.

My nurse bent down to look me in the eye. "You won't be getting any more chemo today — and we'll never give you Taxodere again. We'll get approval for another drug that's easier to take."

After I relaxed a few more minutes, I called Jim at the car repair shop. "Guess what?" I asked. He couldn't guess. I summarized what had just happened.

"I'll be there as soon as I can. I knew I shouldn't have left."

I sighed as I pressed "End" on the cell phone. I would be fine. I just hoped I wouldn't need resuscitation next time.

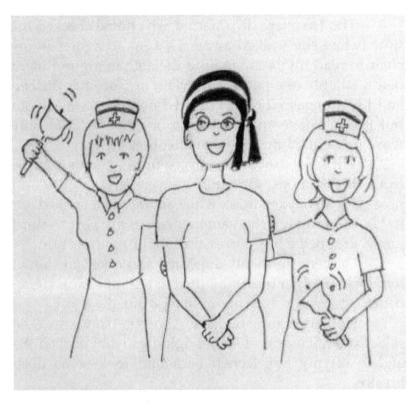

"Hip, hip, hooray! Today is your last day!"

Chapter Ten

Saved by the Belles

February 26, 2019

I made it through the weekend without noticing any after-effects of my allergic reaction to Taxodere on Friday.

I felt well enough to spend some time decorating my house, installing window coverings, making up beds, and putting out towels and cleaning supplies in bathrooms. I had recently received an email from my credit card company listing recent charges, requesting that I verified they were mine. (You know you're overspending when your credit card questions what you're buying. Fortunately, I was through purchasing things for the house for a while.)

The contractors were close to finishing their work, leaving only a few details they would come back for. The house had already been transformed from "dilapidated" to "homey," but there was a lot more to be done. For now, I needed to concentrate on my cancer treatments.

At 8:00 a.m. on Tuesday morning, Jim and I returned to the clinic. This would be my second infusion appointment for what will be my regular schedule if all went well: chemotherapy on two consecutive Tuesdays with one week off, and then back to infusions on consecutive Tuesdays, and a week off and so on, for the next three to four months, depending on how I tolerate it and the results of my blood work and examinations.

As we walked into the reception area, I received a warm welcome from the lady behind the desk. I thought she probably recognized me as the patient they almost killed off three days earlier. Checking me in, she told me we should go first to the waiting room behind her to have my blood dawn for lab work, and then my Nurse Navigator wanted to meet with us.

In short order, I was called in and had my blood drawn that they'd analyze for the doctor to review for my visit with him after chemotherapy.

We then headed back to the administrative offices where Chrissie met us and showed us into her office.

After we were seated, she told us that Dr. Feng had prescribed Abraxane to replace Taxotere and I'd be started on that today.

She went on to explain that the chemical molecules in Abraxane are bound to a protein that makes the drug easier to tolerate. I asked her why I wasn't prescribed Abraxane in the first place if it's preferable.

Chrissy bit her lower lip. "Well, to be honest, the insurance companies want us to try Taxotere first because it's less expensive." Jim and I frowned at each other.

Chrissy continued. "Humana hasn't granted approval for coverage yet for Abraxane, but we've requested an expedited decision. We're expecting to hear any time now."

Jim said, "Any time, meaning…yet this morning? Will Cheryl be getting the drug today? You know, there have been several delays."

Chrissy nodded emphatically. "Absolutely. We've talked to Humana. They know you're here and we're just waiting for the approval to come in. I'm sorry for this inconvenience."

Jim grumbled as we stood to leave. Outside, we made our way down to the waiting area by the Infusion room. Before taking seats for an indeterminate wait, we both got a cup of coffee.

A half hour went by without word. After another half hour Jim said he was going to see what he could find out. When he came back several minutes later, he reported he had found Dr. Feng and urged him to get actively involved in the case. He had also talked to the supervising nurse in Infusion, requesting that she call Humana to get a status report on the Board's review.

She came out a little later to advise that she had called Humana and was told by Authorization that we should be hearing something within the next few minutes.

Finally, at noon we received word that the Board at Humana had voted to approve the payment for Abraxane and were ushered into the chemo room.

I was hooked up to the IV for preliminary meds and steroids which were infused without any ill effect. As the Abraxane drip was started I felt jumpy with anxiety, but the bag emptied without incident. I was then infused with Cytoxan for another hour. I had completed my first round of chemo.

Near the end of my infusion, everyone's attention was drawn to a group of nurses who rang bells and cheered a female patient. A nurse near me explained that this was how they celebrated a patient finishing a course of chemo. I teared up at the woman's happiness, and envisioned my own celebration when I would have completed treatment in a few months.

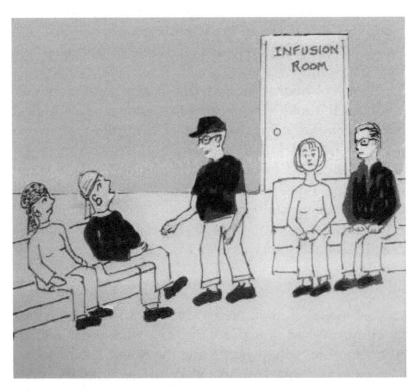

"I'm telling you, it's true. I read it on Facebook."

Chapter Eleven

The Tuesday Chemo Club

March 5, 2019

Turning into the nearly full parking lot of the Tennessee Cancer Specialists the next Tuesday morning, I was reminded of how many people have cancer and are going through the same treatment I am.

I had done some research on the Internet and learned that in the United States, one in two women and one in three men will develop cancer at some point in their lifetime; that one-quarter of new cancer cases are diagnosed in people aged 65 to 74; my age-group.

Doctors explain that the reason cancer seems to be so common nowadays is because people are living longer.

If I could find any good news in the statistics, it was that those with non-metastatic breast cancer like mine have a five-year survival rate of 90%; a ten-year survival rate of 84%. People with other cancers that are easy to diagnose have a survival rate of more than 80% for ten years or more.

I had to stay positive, knowing that the scans, chemotherapy, medications, surgeries, and procedures would help me survive, even if there were hard days ahead when I would have to deal with side effects.

I got out of the car, stretched and inhaled, preparing myself mentally for another round of chemotherapy. I had taken all my pre-treatment drugs to counteract the chemo drugs, and had a drawer-full of medications on hand, if needed, after treatment.

Since my first infusion, I had experienced some fatigue after a couple of days which I dealt with by quitting work on the house by 4:00 in the afternoon.

Inside the clinic, we checked in and took seats near the lab to have my blood drawn.

After that I had a brief consultation with Dr Feng. He was satisfied that I tolerated the Abraxane and Cytoxan to have a second chemotherapy session that day.

As we walked over to the Infusion waiting area and sat down, I smiled and nodded to a couple of ladies I recognized from my last session. They both wore tell-tale scarves turban-style around their heads. I was planning on shopping for a wig soon as I could expect hair loss after three weeks of chemotherapy. Another patient I recognized entered the waiting room and said "hello" to me. I realized I would be seeing the same group of people every week. I had become a regular member of what I thought of as the Tuesday Chemo Club.

Since there were already several people in the waiting room, Jim and I fixed ourselves a cup of coffee from the complimentary urn. I commented to Jim on how weak the coffee was, noting that it's provided for patients before they're infused with poisons.

We sat down to join a group sitting on sofas. One male patient excitedly talked about a report he had heard that insurance companies had stopped paying for Neulasta beyond the first cycle. This was distressing news as we all knew that each dose cost several thousands of dollars.

I would be receiving the drug for the first time that day as it's given on Day 8 of a chemo cycle. The delivery is often by means of a patch that releases the drug within twenty-seven hours to shock bone marrow into manufacturing healthy white and red blood cells to counteract the loss of healthy blood cells by the chemo drugs. Neulasta has several possible bad side effects including severe bone pain and stabbing chest pains.

As the man kept talking, I became more skeptical of his information as he related other problems he had had with insurance companies. I decided to look into the matter on the Internet when I returned home.

My infusion went as well as last Tuesday, finishing off the Abraxane and Cytoxan without ill effects. The nurse came over to apply the Neulasta patch on my right upper arm and to give me instructions.

"After a maximum of twenty-seven hours, you should hear a buzzer go off," she said. "That's the delivery of the medicine that takes about 45 minutes. You can take off the patch when the little tube goes down to zero." I couldn't see the tube, but took her word for it.

She took a breath. "You may experience some side effects tomorrow—like feeling you're having a heart attack, or aching bones, or neuropathy in your hands and feet."

My mouth dropped open.

"These should be temporary," she added. "And not everyone experiences them. Call us if you're running a fever or your pain medication isn't working, okay?"

I nodded, thinking I may want to call an ambulance, instead.

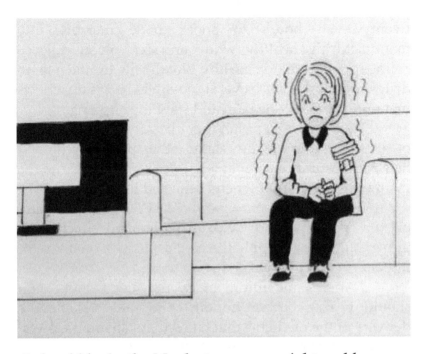

I should be in the Neulasta commercial to add some realism.

Chapter Twelve

Not Playing a Patient on TV

March 6 - 12, 2019

I stayed inside all the next day, not daring to drive the car or even walk away from the house for fear I would have sudden chest pains or an attack of neuropathy in my feet.

My Neulasta buzzer was set to go off by five o'clock p.m. at the latest. At four-thirty I sat on the sofa to watch TV and wait for the signal and whatever physical reaction might follow. Five o'clock came and went without any buzzing or any pain.

I turned down the TV to be sure I could hear my patch going off as I didn't know how loud it would be. By six o'clock, there still hadn't been any buzzing or physical reaction.

Now I was worried that *nothing* had happened. I ran up to my bathroom to look at the gauge on the patch. I twisted my arm and used a hand mirror, but I couldn't get a frontal view to read it.

By seven o'clock I had decided I must have done something wrong and had wasted the expensive drug. Rifling through my Patient Resources Guide, I found the clinic's after-hours emergency number and dialed it. The nurse on duty answered promptly. After I explained the situation, she advised me to rip off the tape to remove the gauge to see it.

While she stayed on the line, I pulled the bandaging off. Nervously, I held the tiny vial up to the light.

"It's on empty," I said, relieved.

"Oh, that's good," she replied. "I think the buzzer simply malfunctioned, but the drug was released on time."

After I hung up, I returned to the sofa to watch some TV to calm down, but as soon as I got comfortable, I saw a Neulasta commercial come on. An attractive woman in her forties sits on a sofa in a doctor's office that morphs into her living room to make the point that the medicine can be infused later in the comfort of your home. Her husband comes in, sits next to her and gives her a hug. Moments later, they get up and stroll out onto their back deck, smiling and holding hands. Their yellow Lab joins them for a game of fetch.

I thought of how *I* had just played out the scene, rigidly sitting on the edge of my sofa, anxiously checking my watch and the patch, then running into the bathroom to contort my arm in the mirror to try to see the gauge, and finally calling an emergency number for medical help. My portrayal wouldn't have sold many on using Neulasta.

The next couple of days I felt okay; at least I didn't have numb feet or achy bones. I kept busy getting my house ready for my brother Bob who was coming to stay overnight before driving us to South Bend to visit relatives. Our Aunt Vernelle was celebrating her 95th birthday. She had recently sold her home and moved into an Independent Living apartment, still enjoying relatively good health. It was a reminder that I came from strong Swedish stock.

On Saturday morning, Bob and I started out in the pouring rain. After about an hour of tense driving with poor vision and heavy truck traffic, the Neulasta suddenly kicked in. As Bob needed to concentrate on his driving, I tried not to let on that I was being riddled with stabbing pains in my lower back and down my legs. Fortunately, they were sporadic, and eased for several minutes between attacks.

It rained without stopping for the entire nine-hour trip. I was relieved when we could finally pull off the road for dinner so I could relax. As soon as we were seated, I felt another sharp pinch in my lower back.

All during weekend my back pains came and went. I was grateful to be distracted by the activity of getting together with my relatives. They took my mind off my discomfort.

Bob and I had good weather on the drive back on Monday and I felt pretty good by the time we arrived at my home. It had been a pleasurable weekend and I was glad I had been able to participate.

That evening my mood darkened when I recalled that I had an appointment at Tennessee Cancer Specialists the first thing the next morning.

I was in a funk when I arrived at the clinic the next day. However, since it was my Tuesday off chemotherapy, I only needed to have my blood drawn. That seemed like a party after enduring my first week on Neulasta.

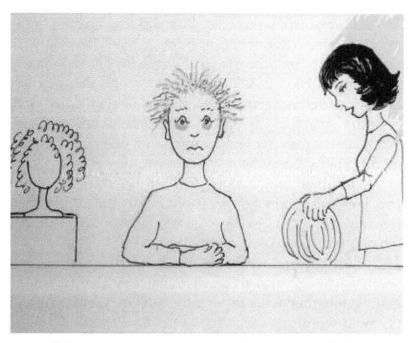

"Here, Mrs. Peyton. Try this on — quick!"

Chapter Thirteen

Getting Wigged Out

March 13-15, 2019

After nearly three weeks of receiving chemotherapy, I hadn't yet begun to lose my hair. Then, one morning I was blow-drying my hair after my shower, using a rounded brush to turn it under, when I noticed the brush was becoming more and more wrapped in hair. By the time I finished, I had enough on my brush to make a Shih Tzu.

Looking at myself in the mirror, I was shocked that my hair was suddenly so thin I could see my scalp. As I pulled on it, strands came off in my hand. I thought I could probably pull out most of my hair right then. It was time to get a wig.

After I dressed and put on makeup using my magnifying mirror, I saw that my eyebrows had thinned and I didn't have many eyelashes. Egads, I was going to look like an egg.

When I put on my foundation, I did find a few new hairs—above my lip and on my chin. It appeared that the only place I could still grow hair was where I didn't want it.

A couple days later, Jim and I stopped at a wig store where I had previously bought small hair pieces I clipped onto my own hair when I pulled it back. This would be a much more significant purchase as I would be wearing the wig every day for several months. That day I wrapped a bandana around my head as a cover-up.

Upon entering the store, Jim stood back while I walked up and down the aisles, looking over the dozens of wigs they carried in all colors and styles. Unfortunately, I didn't see one that was at all similar to what my own blonde hair had looked like. Most of the wigs were dark-colored, made of Dynel, and were thicker and shinier than natural hair. My hair had been fine and straight. I usually wore it chin-length and turned under. I wanted to look as much like myself as possible.

Having seen everything on display, I stopped one of the saleswomen to ask if they had any other wigs. "Oh, yes," she said. "We have a whole stockroom full in the back. What are you looking for?"

As I explained my situation, she nodded and smiled, telling me that they had many chemotherapy clients and suggested we follow her to the back where I could sit at one of their dressing tables and she'd bring me wigs from their stock.

As I sat down facing a three-sided mirror, I removed my bandana and she examined what little hair I still had.

"I'm sure we'll find something," she said, probably thinking it was an emergency. "Let me go to the back and bring out a few for you to try."

A few minutes later she returned with several plastic bags full of wigs. I was pleased that she had been observant, bringing out several possibilities. All of them were thicker and had more body than my hair had ever had, but they were of a similar color and were my style and length.

I tried them on using a hand mirror to see the back of each one. It came down to two choices. Trying one on and then the other, I asked Jim which he liked better. He chose the one I was leaning towards.

"How much?" he asked. I looked at the price sticker and was pleasantly surprised to see that it was under $150.00; a good price for a quality wig.

As we left the store, I felt that people who knew me wouldn't think I looked all that different in the wig.

The weather was unseasonably warm the next day making me anxious to start planting in the bare dirt in front of my house where the old landscaping materials had been removed weeks earlier.

Putting on my wig, I drove out to a nearby nursery and picked up a few shrubs.

It was quite windy by the time I got home and started digging. As I was bending and standing, I could feel my wig shifting, with some hair blowing across my face. I was reluctant to brush them aside as I could envision the wig catching an updraft and taking off with me chasing it around the neighborhood.

I went inside and put on a hat as a precaution. Wearing a hat over a wig feels pretty much like you're wearing a helmet, but it gave me a feeling of security.

As time went on, I would discover other downsides of wearing a wig — like it being too warm, itching, and giving me a headache; but I was always grateful that it allowed me to go out in public looking normal with a decent head of hair.

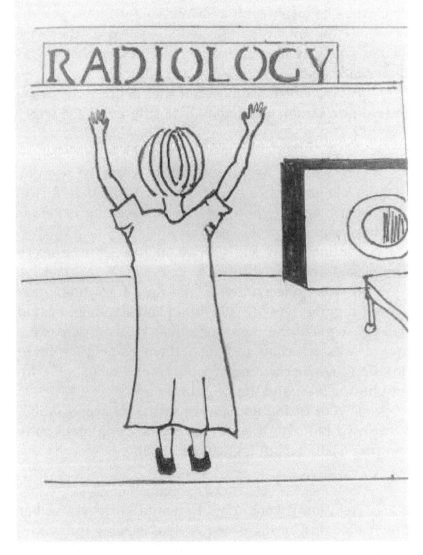

"Hey, everybody! Guess who's back!"

Chapter Fourteen

Another Day, Another CT Scan

March 19, 2019

On the third Tuesday in March, Jim and I arrived at the cancer clinic at 10:00 a.m. for my weekly appointment. My routine was to first have my blood drawn for lab analysis, then see Dr Feng or his Nurse Practitioner for a consultation, and finally to be infused with chemotherapy with the other members of the Tuesday Chemo Club.

Soon after I checked in and made my $40 co-payment, we headed toward the lab waiting room, stopping along the way to get a cup of water. When I pulled the bottom cup down from the dispenser, the whole stack broke loose and tumbled to the floor, rolling off in every direction. I quickly collected and restacked them before anyone saw me. I hoped this wasn't an omen on how the day would go.

I had only gulped down half a glass of water before I heard my name called to report for blood work. The nurse efficiently accessed my port and drew my blood, filling three vials. Maybe the rest of the day would go smoothly.

We next met with Dr. Feng's Nurse Practitioner in an examining room, she took my vitals as I sat in one of the chairs. No problem. She inquired about my reactions to the Neulasta infusion the past week. I replied that I had suffered episodes of sharp pains in my lower back and down my legs that had eased after a while. She didn't seem surprised or concerned about my report since the side effects I described were commonplace.

She then pressed the subject, asking I had experienced any other ill effects. Thinking back, I recalled that I had been short of breath whenever I exerted myself, like taking the dog for a walk up the hills in my neighborhood. She raised her eyebrows at this. Stepping over to a cabinet, she brought back a stethoscope and listened to my lungs. Without commenting on what she had heard, she told us she'd be back shortly with the doctor. Closing the door behind her, she left us questioning whether there was a problem.

She soon returned with Dr. Feng who greeted me effusively and shook my hand. After a few pleasantries, he sat on a corner of the examining table. Jutting out his lower lip, he nodded curtly. "We need you to have a CT scan before your treatment." He waved away my look of surprise. "Just of your chest. It's possible you have blood clot."

He went on to tell me that a clot would require treatment before I could resume chemotherapy.

The nurse added that she had already notified the radiation department at Parkwest to work me in so I could return for treatment that day if I didn't have a "PE" (pulmonary embolism).

Jim and I sighed as we gathered our things together to prepare to leave for the hospital.

A few minutes later we pulled up to the entrance and left the car with the valet service. Inside, we checked in at the front desk, then waited for my registration interview when I was asked for a co-pay of $200, which I hadn't expected.

After signing the paperwork, we headed over to the out-patient waiting room and took our regular seats closest to the TV. The set was tuned to HGTV, as always. An episode of "Fixer Upper" was on.

In about twenty minutes, I was called in, (missing the reveal of the redone house). In an examining room I had to wait for a technician to come and hook me up to an IV. It took another twenty minutes for the radiation room to become available. Finally, I was brought to the CT room and positioned on the cot by the scanner.

The abbreviated procedure took just a few minutes and I returned to the small interior waiting room.

A half hour later the technician appeared again to tell me I could go back to the clinic where my doctor would review the results with me. I gave him a questioning look.

In response he said, "I can't go over everything with you, but I can tell you that you don't have a blood clot."

I returned to the outpatient waiting room and told Jim the good news. We hurried back to the clinic, hoping there was enough time for me to be infused.

I was the last patient of the day, quickly hooked up to an IV drip, and left to settle back for the two hours it would take to empty the three bags of solution.

Dr. Feng came out waving my CT report. "Not to worry," he said. "It's just an infection. You take anti-biotic for eight days and we'll see." He patted me on the shoulder and left.

We started for home at 4:00 p.m. as the clinic was closing. It had been a six-hour appointment and had cost me an additional $240, but at least I didn't have a blood clot. What will they think of next?

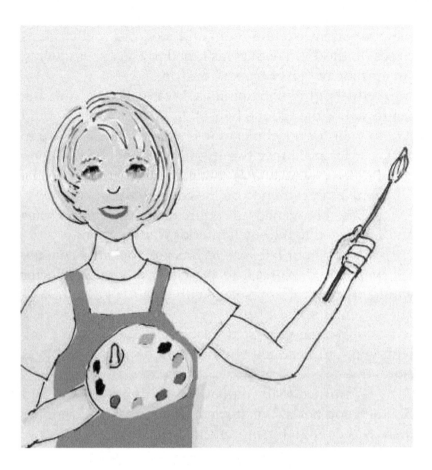

"Painting is the best medicine."

Chapter Fifteen

Patient Turned Painter

March 26 – April 6, 2019

When I checked into the cancer clinic for my regular appointment on the last Tuesday in March, the receptionist told me I didn't need to see the doctor or nurse practitioner that day since my chemo treatments had been going so well. Until further notice, I would be scheduled for only blood drawings and infusions.

This was the first really good news I had received since starting chemotherapy. I felt a little cocky as I started back to the Infusions waiting room, smiling smugly as I passed the lounge for those who had to see the doctor.

I took a seat on one of the sofas near the door to the chemo room and picked up a periodical to flip through to pass the time. It was titled, "Guide to Metastatic Breast Cancer." Maybe "People" or "Time" would have been better distractions in a cancer clinic?

At least the feature article, "Four Years Later I'm Here, I'm Hopeful, and I'm Happy" had a good ending.

When I was called in, my usual chair nearest the nurses' station was taken, but I figured with my new status I could chance being a little further away.

I found a chair in the last row, close to the snack table. Looking around, I didn't recognize the people in the area since most people take the same chair each time. The middle-aged man on my left must have been a regular the way he managed to stand in one motion and then smoothly guided his IV stand across the room to get a snack. I hadn't tried walking with my stand yet.

The women near me appeared to be at various stages of treatment. One frail older woman with a bald head was curled up under a blanket, while a younger, sturdy-looking woman sat bolt upright, engrossed in a book. A third woman was covered up in sweats and a ski cap under a thick lap robe.

I always wore my best casual clothes and my wig for my appointments to make myself feel and look better.

Following my infusion with steroids and Abraxane, my nurse taped the Neulasta patch onto the back of my right arm and told me I could leave. It was just 11:00. I'd been there for only one hour; a record.

I felt fine for the rest of the day and evening, but knew that any side effects wouldn't be apparent until after three o'clock the next day when the Neulasta was released into my blood stream.

I rested most of the next day feeling depressed and lacking energy. A little after 3:00, my patch buzzed, signifying the injection of the drug, but no pains followed.

I was still pain-free on Thursday, but I couldn't shake the melancholy and the feeling of lack of purpose. To bring myself out of the funk, I decided to work on a creative project on the front of the house. I had already painted the gutters, soffit, garage door, and trim, but I wanted to so some trompe l'œil (French for "fool the eye") painting of stones on the cedar boards under the long windows that would match the real stones on the front of the house.

Mixing my artists' oil paints in the various colors of the stones, I finished my project in a few hours.

Two neighbors walking by were amazed how real the stones looked. They lifted my spirits.

Not having an appointment at the cancer clinic the following Tuesday, I spent the next week on home improvements to stay positive and to keep up my energy.

I first went to the local hardware store and bought a couple flats of impatiens to plant in front. When I pushed my cart over to the counter to pay, the woman in front of me turned and glared at my flowers. "You can't plant those before April 25th," she snapped.

I offered the obvious defense. "They're selling them now."

The woman was not to be deterred. "They want you to come back and buy more after they die."

Jeesh, what a sourpuss. I was like a Pollyanna compared to her.

The next day I decided to decorate my garage door with carriage-style trim: strap hinges, handles, and "windows." I drove into town to the Home Depot where I bought the hardware and a jar of black exterior paint.

At home I went right to work, marking places for the hinges and center handle, then drilling and attaching everything with screws. Finally, I created the faux carriage windows by measuring and masking off four "panes," for each of eight windows, and brushing on the glossy black paint,

When I finished, I ran out to the street to view the effect. It looked like the real thing — even to me.

That evening I thought about how my work had energized me and made me feel more positive. That lesson would serve me well in the coming months of treatment. I was already anxious to start painting bricks on the driveway.

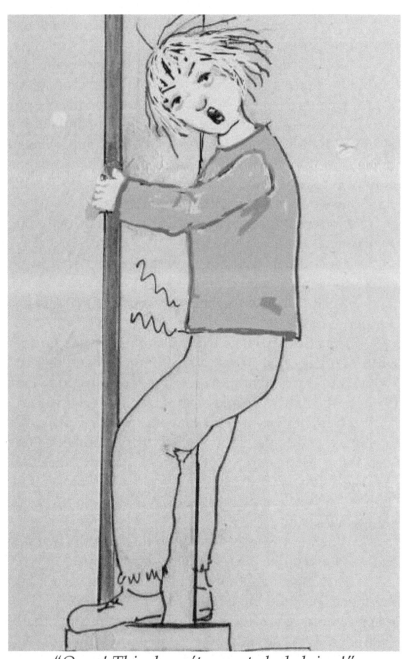

"Oww! This doesn't seem to be helping!"

Chapter Sixteen

From Faux Stones to Kidney Stones

April 9 - 13, 2019

Within a couple days after finishing my faux painting and garage door, I suffered an unexpected health crisis that would send me to the emergency room.

My Tuesday Chemo Club went well enough, although we had longer wait times than usual. After having my blood drawn for lab work, I was scheduled to see Dr. Feng for a routine consultation. Since he was backed up with patients, Jim and I had a long wait both out front and in the examination room.

When Dr. Feng finally came in, he said I looked well, briefly went over my blood work which was satisfactory, and asked how I had handled the Neulasta. He was happy to hear that I hadn't had side effects this time. After a few encouraging remarks, he sent me off to report for chemotherapy.

The treatment room was nearly filled with patients and visitors. Fortunately, Jim and I were able to find a recliner and guest chair near the snack cart, which was our new favorite location. They often had homemade treats along with packaged cookies and bars that we liked to sample with our coffee or cold drinks.

Since we were sitting in close proximity to several other patients and guests, I could overhear several of their conversations and observe their interactions. I was struck by how pleasant and kind everyone was.

One patient's wife crossed the aisle to visit with an elderly woman who sat by herself. In the conversation, I learned that the patient was ninety-years old and had been coming to the clinic for several years for intravenous B-12 treatments to boost her immune system. Her daughter would be coming to pick her up.

A feeble-looking old man was accompanied by a male friend of about the same age who kept up a lively conversation that the patient seemed to enjoy during the entire treatment time.

I observed how cheerful and attentive the nurses were; always happy to bring over beverages, blankets, or magazines to the patients.

In all my time at the clinic, I never heard anyone be rude or complain. It was inspiring how everyone made the best of the situation.

By the time I was finished that day, Jim and I had been at the clinic for over four hours, but I felt the time had been well spent.

* * *

Two days later I started experiencing sharp abdominal cramps. At first, I wasn't too concerned since I often had aches and pains following treatment. Rummaging through my stock of drugs I found some pills to counteract pain.

By Friday afternoon, the cramping had worsened. I took another pill and curled up in a ball to hold in the pain, pulling a blanket around me.

Thankfully, by evening the pains had subsided. I thought they must have been a temporary reaction to my latest round of chemotherapy.

I was awakened early Saturday morning with severe abdominal cramps and hobbled downstairs to call the cancer clinic's emergency number. When a nurse answered, I breathlessly explained my condition. She prescribed two over-the-counter medications and urged me to call back if I didn't get relief.

I called Jim to pick up the pills. Hearing my shaky voice, he said he'd get them and be right over.

By the time he arrived fifteen minutes later, I was outside, wrapped around a post on my porch trying to get relief from the intense pain. Jim jumped out of the car and insisted we go to the hospital. I didn't argue. The pain was so severe I could barely breathe.

At the hospital, the registration lady rushed me through the paperwork while I squirmed and moaned in my chair. After I signed whatever documents were necessary, she called for a gurney and aides whisked me back to the emergency room. The doctor on duty examined me, feeling around my abdomen while I bit my lip trying not to cry out. Within a few minutes I was hooked up to an IV of Dilaudid, a strong opioid, that cut through the pain to make it bearable.

I was taken down to radiology for a CT scan that revealed a kidney stone in my bladder. The doctor explained that my pain had been caused by the stone moving down one of the 8"– 10" ureters from the kidney. He predicted I would undergo more pain to pass it.

After a couple of hours I was released home with Percocet to take for the final passage. I wasn't looking forward to the trip.

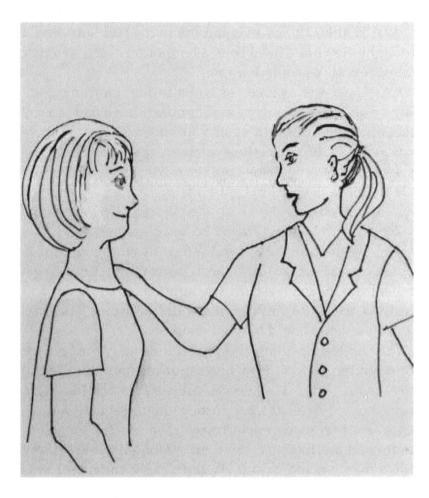

"I feel your pain . . . level."

Chapter Seventeen

No Pain, No Gain

April 17, 2019

The Tuesday Chemo Club the next week was unusually abbreviated. I wasn't scheduled to see Dr. Feng, and my infusion was cut back to my pre-meds and Abraxane, finishing with the Neulasta patch on my arm. I finally understood that *none* of the Neulasta was released until after it had been on my arm for 24 hours and the mechanism had pinged. I had been staying home the whole next day after getting the patch, nervously awaiting horrendous bone pain. I could have been working.

It looked like it was a day off for most of the clinic patients, with fewer than ten people spread out among the five rows of recliners. The only patient near my seat (closest to the snack table) was a diminutive, elderly Asian man who slept soundly under a lap robe drawn up to his chin. His equally petite wife sat by him, keeping watch, her legs crossed demurely at the ankles. They struck me as being the picture of quiet dignity.

Since my assigned nurse was not busy with other patients that day, I took the opportunity of extra time with her to relate the story of my recent kidney stone attack. In describing the pain, I made a comparison to the pain of a ruptured appendix I had suffered years earlier when I was rushed into surgery in the middle of the night to save my life. My conclusion was that the kidney stone pain was worse and I was still waiting for the stone to pass.

While I was relating the details of my kidney stone attacks, my nurse was listening with rapt attention and nodding with understanding.

When I was finished, she told me that she too had experienced the agony of having a kidney stone, and had been taken to the nearest emergency room reeling in agony.

As she described the pain as being excruciating, I felt justified in saying that it was the worst pain imaginable, considering that a nurse probably has a higher pain threshold than most people and doesn't use hyperbole in describing it.

She had passed her kidney stone at that time, and claimed that the pain wasn't worse when it passed than when it had moved down from the kidney to the bladder. I guess that was good news, although it was hard to imagine worse pain.

I left the clinic feeling pretty good and continued being pain-free at home for the rest of the day. I was grateful to not feel effects from the chemotherapy as well as having relief from the pain of the kidney stone that was still lying in wait to attack me.

Sure enough, at six o'clock the next morning I was awakened by agonizing pain in my lower left side. I curled myself into a protective ball, hoping the spasm would soon pass. I felt if I moved at all, even by breathing too deeply, the pain would worsen. After several minutes, I thought the pain had even intensified and I needed to take one of the drugs the emergency room doctor had prescribed.

I rolled out of bed, still hunched over and holding my side. Staying in this position, I clambered downstairs to the kitchen and rifled through my medicine drawer looking for the oxycodone, the strongest drug I had.

Finding the bottle, I took one out and swallowed it, then wrote down the time as 6:15. I would have to wait three hours before it was safe to take another one, and I had to judge the intensity carefully as I had only twelve pills.

By a quarter to seven the drug had miraculously knocked out the pain. It was easy for me to understand how someone could get addicted to taking opioids.

Later that morning when I was out walking my dog, Cody, I felt another stirring of discomfort. I told him if he had to do "business," he'd better do it quickly. He must have understood because he cooperated for a change, and we hurried home. By the time we walked inside, the uneasiness was gone.

But by five o'clock the pain had returned, full-force. Since I hadn't taken another oxycodone during the day, I didn't hesitate to take one then, hoping I'd have relief again in a half hour. Right on schedule, by 5:30 the pain had gone away and I felt good enough to start putting something together for dinner.

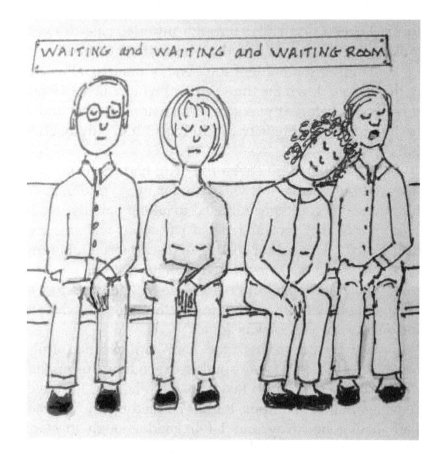

Chapter Eighteen

The Waiting Game

April 24, 2019

I didn't have Tuesday Chemo Club the third week of April, but did manage to have a doctor's appointment in the Parkwest hospital tower.

On Wednesday of that week I saw the urologist for a second time to check on my kidney stone. I didn't think I had passed it, but wasn't sure, so the doctor gave me a little netted scoop to hold onto during every bathroom visit. That seemed too unpleasant, so I kept it handy, but not in my hand.

As Jim and I approached the elevator in the Tower a little before ten, I remarked that this appointment shouldn't be a repeat of the last one that had taken two hours, mostly spent sitting in the waiting room.

But, when we got upstairs and saw how many people were there ahead of us, we weren't encouraged that we'd have a better outcome. The room looked like a passenger gate inside an airport when it was close to take-off time. We had to make our way around three rows of people to nab the last two vacant chairs that were together.

After we were seated, I stashed my purse under my chair and looked around to gauge how long the wait could be. After deducting those I took for spouses, I counted seventeen patients to see the one doctor. I didn't need to do the math to know that we were looking at over an hour's wait.

When no one had been called in the first fifteen minutes, I walked over to the check-in desk to ask for some information about the wait time.

The receptionist looked up at me without expression. "Uh, the doctor is running about a half-hour late," she said, matter-of-factly.

Just a half hour? I made a show of scanning the crowd, then looked back at her, widening my eyes in disbelief.

"Some are here for blood tests or imaging," she offered as an explanation for her prediction of a relatively short wait time. It seemed like too many blood tests for one group of people, but I couldn't refute the statement.

I went back to my seat, picking up a magazine on my way. I flipped through it for a while then, bored, I closed my eyes.

I was half-asleep when Jim nudged me that I was being called by the doctor's nurse. It was eleven-thirty; an hour and a half after our appointment time. Jim grumbled under his breath that we were the last people in the waiting room. As I stood, I felt a little shaky.

We followed the nurse back to an examining room for the usual preliminary interview and procedures. After taking my blood pressure, she frowned as she announced, "It's 104 over 60. Are you being treated for low blood pressure?"

I told her my pressure was normally low, but I did feel a little light-headed right then. I explained that I was on a course of chemotherapy and needed to eat something every three to four hours and I hadn't had anything since early morning. She nodded and said she'd get me an energy bar. That should help, I thought.

She returned a minute later and set down a granola bar in front of me. As I reached for it, she put her hand out. "Oh, don't eat it until the doctor sees you. He might want to operate this afternoon."

She left me to look longingly at the treat, wondering why the doctor would want to operate on me without any new information or preparation.

Ten minutes later the doctor came in with the film of my CT scan from my emergency room visit. As he held it up, I thought of the old urology joke where the doctor tells the patient, "I looked at your kidney stone test. You didn't pass."

I was then asked to get up on the table and lay back while the doctor pressed on my lower abdomen. I told him it was uncomfortable, but not painful.

He asked me how I had been the past week and I informed him about my painful episodes that had been managed with the oxycodone. Hearing this, he wrote out a prescription for more pain killers and said I should make an appointment to come back in a week for a recheck, assuming I would pass the stone. If I didn't pass it in the next day or two, he would schedule surgery for May 2, eight days from then, to "break up" the stone.

Jim and I stopped at the front desk for me to make an appointment for the next Wednesday. I commented that I was the last patient in the place, adding that I had never waited so long to see a doctor.

She gave a little shrug of unconcern. "I don't know how that happened today."

I turned to roll my eyes, thinking, *How about over-scheduling as an explanation?*

As Jim got the door for me, I ripped open my then flattened protein bar and took a bite.

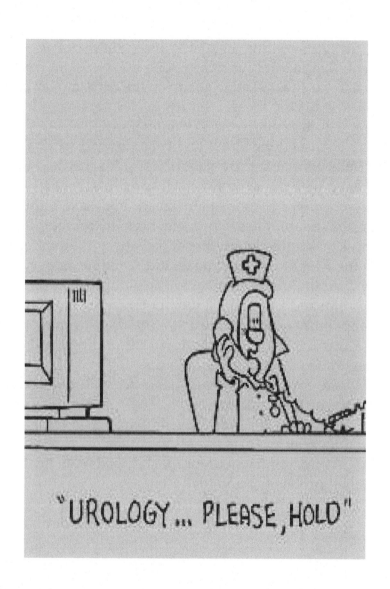

Chapter Nineteen

Having a Surgery I Can't Pronounce

April 26 – May 2, 2019

Since I hadn't knowingly passed the stone by the following Friday, I called the urologist's office in the late morning to let them know. They said they'd call back to confirm my surgery for the following Thursday, May 2. I had learned the procedure was called a ureteroscopy lithotripsy. I hoped I wouldn't have to say that when I checked in at the hospital.

Not hearing anything by the afternoon, I called the office again, knowing they'd be closed over the weekend. I was advised they still hadn't gotten a confirmation. This urology group didn't rush into anything.

I called the office for the third time at 5:00 p.m. A recorded message advised that the office was closed and to call back Monday morning. No alternate number. I needed to know before Monday in order to discontinue the drug Warfarin for five to seven days before the procedure as I had been advised. Now what?

Fortunately, I could call the cancer clinic's off-hours phone number and consult with them. The nurse who answered assured me I could safely discontinue Warfarin before my chemo therapy on Tuesday, but it was essential I discontinue it for the surgery on Thursday.

Okay. I could get ready for surgery, but was it even scheduled? Surprisingly, on Sunday afternoon my urologist left a message on our my answering machine that my surgery was set for Thursday and I should come to the hospital at 9:00 a.m. to prep for the procedure at 11:00. And don't forget to discontinue the Warfarin. Thanks.

On Tuesday, the staff at the cancer clinic asked me about my intended surgery later that week to determine if I could receive any treatment. Luckily, I had all the details of the procedure on my phone from the "Urology Portal," (of all names). Dr. Feng was relieved to learn that the surgery would be done with a scope and not by incision so I could have my chemotherapy.

Making our way through the infusion room, Jim and I took seats near the snack table. That morning someone had brought in homemade "pink lemonade cupcakes" for the patients. They were delicious and a special treat to make the infusion time more pleasant.

Later, at home, I received a call from Parkwest that I needed to come in on Wednesday for pre-testing and registration prior to my surgery. My co-pay would be $225 for the hospital, and I'd be billed separately by the doctor and anesthesiologist. I called Humana to confirm my costs, and was elated to learn that I had met my maximum out-of-pocket costs of $3,400 as of March 30. I wouldn't owe anything more for the rest of the year!

On the day of my procedure, nick-named "tripsy" for good reason, the oncologist's office called us at home at 8:00 a.m. to see if we could get on our way right then. There had been a cancellation and I could be seen earlier than planned.

Just as we pulled up at the hospital, my cell phone ring tone sounded. The office was calling again to see if we had arrived as they were ready for me. Geez. I hoped they'd wait long enough to anesthetize me.

The next hour was spent getting me ready for surgery. First, I was wheeled through a rabbit warren of rooms and corridors to get to my assigned room where I changed into an open sleeveless smock. Then I was taken out for a quick x-ray, and back to "my room" for vitals and an IV hook-up. My anesthesiologist popped in to introduce himself and asked if I had any problems with anesthesia. (Hospital personnel are like courtroom lawyers—they only ask questions they already know the answers to.)

The next thing I remember was waking up in a recovery room in a row of beds occupied by patients who were looking around in confusion like I was. Somehow, I had on my own clothes again. A nurse approached and told me I was ready to go home. She helped me into a wheelchair and off we went, backtracking the original route.

When I saw Jim in the waiting room, he told me the procedure went well except that the kidney stone wasn't in my bladder to be blasted. It was gone. I must have passed it during one of my painful episodes. I wondered why that wasn't known from the X-ray that morning; but . . . whatever. I was just glad to go home in my groggy state to recuperate.

Before we left, the doctor came out to talk to us. He explained that they can only confirm the presence of a kidney stone in an X-ray, but they can't confirm its absence if they don't see it. That actually made sense to me. Of course, I might have still been under the influence of the anesthetic.

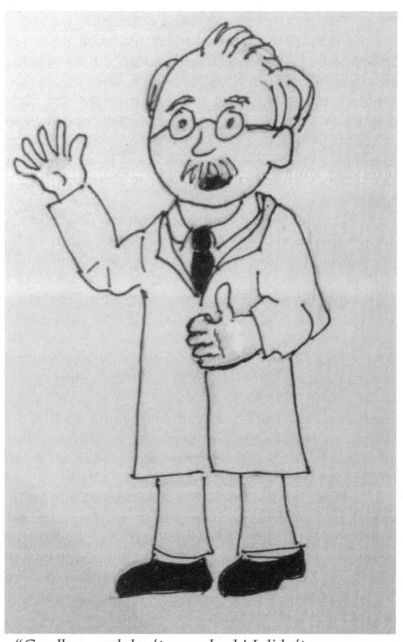

"Goodbye, and don't come back! I didn't mean you, Mrs. Peyton."

Chapter Twenty

A Second Invader Leaves

May 3, 2019

I missed my appointment at the cancer clinic the first Tuesday in May. When I should have been there, sitting in a recliner and hooked up to an IV, I was on my hands and knees in my backyard digging out poison ivy. Why? Besides the fact that the weed is unsightly and a menace, I was confused as to what week it was, thinking it was my "off week."

The previous Tuesday Dr. Feng had made a point of telling me that I needed to get a mammogram during my week off to check on the size of the tumor after completing three cycles of chemotherapy. I left, thinking I understood him to mean the *next week*, (although I had a printed schedule with the right dates).

After working all Tuesday morning in the heat, I felt sweaty and itchy and came inside at eleven o'clock to shower and throw my clothes in the laundry.

Before I had a chance to do that, I received a phone call from the cancer clinic. They were looking for me because I was an hour late for my treatment. I was embarrassed I had missed my regular time after being in a routine for over two months. I had heard about people in treatment getting "chemo brain," which was having decreased memory, but I knew I had just been careless and couldn't blame that on the drugs.

I thanked the clinic worker for calling and apologized for my oversight and promised I wouldn't miss my next appointment. She encouraged me to come in that afternoon so I wouldn't get off my schedule; that they would work me in, no problem. Like everyone who works at the clinic, she only wanted to be helpful and not to place blame. As I hung up, I thought that, for a group of people who spent their days poisoning patents, they were really very nice.

When I arrived at the clinic at 1:30 p.m., the nursing staff seemed glad to see me and graciously dismissed my apologies as being unnecessary. They pointed out that it was my "short" day so my treatment wouldn't take much time.

After my blood was drawn for labs, I was infused with steroids and Abraxane. My nurse then taped the Neulasta patch on my arm and told me I was all set to go home. I didn't need to consult with Dr. Feng.

The patch was scheduled to go off and start injecting the drug at around 6:30 that night. After that I'd wait to see if I had any serious reactions, which I didn't expect, since I had tolerated the drug several previous times.

When I got home, I called the Comprehensive Breast Center to make an appointment for a mammogram the following week. They had an opening on Friday which I took. I was anxious to see how effective chemotherapy had been in reducing the size of the tumor. Maybe it had simply disappeared like my kidney stone. I thought of the song from "*The Sound of Music:*" "Farewell, So Long, Auf Wiederschen, Good Night; and the Gloria Gaynor song, "I Will Survive."

Friday was 'good news' day. After I had my mammogram at the Center, the radiologist came into my examining room to tell me that my tumor was much smaller than it had been three months earlier.

"It's barely there," he said, surprised at how much it had shrunk. He credited the new chemo drugs like Abraxane for the result. He then congratulated me for doing so well, and told me that I looked really good for someone on chemo. (Not sure if that was a compliment.)

The second good news that day was that I had finally figured out the itchy red rash that came and went on my arms and legs was a side effect of Neulasta. That was why you were prescribed Clariten to take the morning after wearing the patch. I bought some Gold Bond lotion on my way home for some additional relief.

The final good news was from Home Depot. When I stopped to buy color stain for my driveway and patio, the man in the paint department advised me that all the concrete paint and stain would be as going on sale on the 16th of the month for $10 off per gallon. I thanked him for being considerate of their customers. (It probably helped that I was a regular at the paint department and would probably be there on the 16th anyway.)

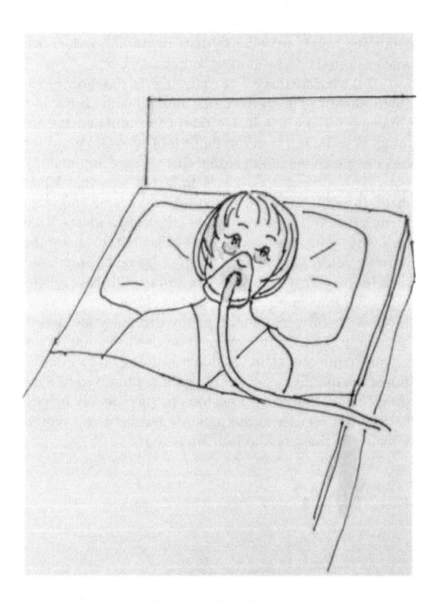

Not my best look.

Chapter Twenty-one

Saving my Breath

May 20 – 22, 2019

A couple of weeks after receiving the good report that the tumor in my right breast had shriveled, my "Neulasta rash" flared up again on my arms and legs, becoming unbearable. The red, bumpy skin had become crusty and bloody, as I couldn't stop scratching. I had started promising myself I could have an ice cream bar if I didn't scratch for 'x' number of hours. Unfortunately, I didn't get many ice cream bars that way.

Becoming desperate for relief, I slathered on every lotion I could find — Hydrocortisone, Calamine, Gold Bond, Solar-Caine; all to no avail.

I tried splashing cold water on my arms and legs during the day and soaking in an oatmeal bath in the evening. I still couldn't bend my elbows without feeling a stabbing pain.

On the third day of this torture I called the cancer clinic to ask if they could recommend something stronger. They called my drug store with a prescription for prednisone which I picked up that day. After downing six pills at once (as allowed), I finally felt some relief.

By the fourth day, I was hopeful that I could control the itching with prednisone, although I couldn't be on the drug for too long.

That evening I noticed I had come down with a sore throat, so I sucked on a couple of lozenges. By the next morning, I had developed a bad cough and my breathing was labored.

That afternoon I thought I was well enough to etch the driveway with chemicals to prepare it for painting. In retrospect, it was evidence that I may have had "chemo brain" after all.

The next morning, a Saturday, I rested and nursed my worsening cold with over-the-counter medications. They didn't seem to be doing much good as I felt miserable, never leaving the couch all day.

By Sunday morning my breathing had become painful and my cough had deepened. I knew by then it wasn't just a cold. I called Jim who said he'd come over right away to drive me to the Emergency room at Fort Loudoun Medical Center, our nearest hospital.

Within the hour we were seated at the registration desk in the emergency room, the same place where I had been a month earlier doubled over in pain from a kidney stone.

After a short wait that seemed long, an orderly came out and escorted us back to one of the chilly examining rooms just off the central nurses' station in the busy department. I undressed down to the waist and put on a cotton gown, then climbed into the single bed that was made up with only a sheet. Thankfully, a nurse soon brought me a heated blanket.

A Dr. Garmon came in with a nurse. Over the next twenty minutes they recorded my medical history, took my vitals taken, listened to my chest, and drew blood. I was then hooked up to a saline IV.

Two aides wheeled in an X-ray machine to take a picture of my chest. More radiation? I thought with all I'd had lately I wouldn't need to be charming to light up a room.

Jim and I then waited anxiously for Dr. Garmon to come back with a diagnosis. I was sure I had pneumonia which I had been hospitalized with twice before.

When the doctor came in, he informed us that I didn't have pneumonia, but had a bronchial infection along with an elevated white blood cell count. Okay, that wasn't good. He said he was admitting me as I would need antibiotics and a ventilator. We would have to wait there until a room was ready.

Jim and I spent the next four hours sitting in the little examining room waiting to hear.

Finally, a nurse came in with a wheelchair to transfer me to the room I'd be staying in. Jim had to leave for a while to take care of the dog.

I was then wheeled down several corridors to a double room on the first floor, where I was assigned to bed 2 by the window. Since I had anticipated being admitted, I had brought an overnight bag with personal effects which I stowed in one of the two empty lockers.

Since I was already in a gown, I got into bed and pulled up the blanket, prepared to be a hospital patient again.

A copy of the Fort Loudoun Medical Center Guidebook had been left on the tray table. Picking it up, I read the first couple of pages that set forth the hospital's philosophy of giving the best patient care available through the use of "state-of the-art equipment and a dedicated medical staff." You could be assured that your medical team would work in tandem on a treatment plan in order for you to fully recover. (Unless you didn't).

I also read in the Guidebook that, in hospitals, "round" is a verb, as in "We will round you every two hours at night" (That's a quote.) Somehow that didn't sound desirable in more ways than one.

I put aside the magazine when I smelled food and noticed that it was dinner time. Using the dining services extension on the phone by my bed, I called to request a dinner tray. Given a few choices, I selected "chopped steak." I figured that was safe, along with potatoes and peas and lemon meringue pie for dessert.

When a cafeteria worker brought up my tray, I dove into it, realizing I hadn't eaten since breakfast. The chopped steak was pretty good and the lemon meringue pie reminded me of my grandmother's, and that's a compliment.

Jim came in after I had finished my dinner. I told him I could order a guest meal for him for the next night. The charge was a modest $5.00. He thought that was a good idea. I told him I'd call when I had the menu that changed with daily specials.

After he left, I was "rounded" several times during the evening by nurses who took my vitals and listened to my lungs. One inserted an IV of erythromycin, then came back a few times to chart the results. At some point Dr. Garmon popped in to tell me he was watching my white blood count and felt sure I would be improving soon.

By eleven o'clock I was exhausted, turned off my light, and fell right to sleep. Sometime afterwards I was awakened by hearing my name being called. Although my room was dark, I could make out two nurses who were backlit from the hall light. They were pushing a large machine toward my bed. I knew I was being rounded again.

The nurses removed a glass panel from the machine and slipped it behind my back, telling me they were taking a chest x-ray.

"What time is it?" I couldn't help but ask.

"Five o'clock," one of them responded without explanation or apology.

After my X-ray, I fell back to sleep, but was soon awakened by more roundings following one another in quick succession. One female nurse came in at 6:00 a.m. to take vitals. A male nurse brought in a ventilator at 6:30 a.m. and had me inhale Albuterol for several minutes to "open my airways." It was a mist that tasted like the ocean that was very disagreeable, especially before the sun came up.

At 7:00, my CNA (Certified Nursing Assistant), came in to write down the names of the staff who would be attending me that day on the white board across from the end of my bed.

Within the next couple of hours, I was visited by the first shift RN, my case manager, the floor doctor, the charge nurse, and the cleaning man. (I swear.)

By the end of the morning, I had had more visitors than I've had at some of my parties.

The kitchen called at 7:30 to ask what I wanted for lunch and dinner. In the Guidebook I had seen lists of entrees, sides, salads, and desserts that are always available, noting additional specials for each day. Since I hadn't read through the list, I had to rush my order and then second-guessed myself later. Would the grilled chicken salad have been better than the cottage cheese and fresh fruit plate? I wondered.

With the list in hand, I called Jim to see what he'd like for dinner. We both decided to pass on the pork chop entrée and go with the stir-fried chicken. I suggested that he order a piece of fruit he could take home, but he thought that was taking unfair advantage. We both selected a dessert. No sense passing up some delicious baked item we'd never have at home.

The next day I got a roommate — an elderly woman who had come up from recovery after having some minor surgery. She was quite talkative, telling me about her friends at the nursing home and her family that lived in the area. Due to her surgery, she wasn't able to move around so I helped out by operating the bed controls for her and retrieving the TV remote and the call button when they slipped between the bed rails.

The next two days became routine. Every hour someone would come in and either perform a test or just see if I needed anything.

One test was to check on my oxygen level. I was able to see on their screen that my number was always 90. I thought that must be pretty good (it would be an "A" in school.) When I asked about it, the nurse replied drolly that I was one point away from wearing an oxygen mask. Oh.

On one visit my oxygen slipped down to 89. The nurse told me to breathe deeply in and out to try to bring up the number. When the level came up to 91, she nodded approvingly and suggested that I occasionally walk down the hallway to increase my oxygen level with exercise. I guess I couldn't just stay in bed and be waited on for three days.

One other concern for the nurses was finding a good vein for my IV. As they explained it, chemotherapy weakens the walls of the veins which caused a few of mine to "blow up," leaking antibiotic into my tissues that hurt like the dickens. One nurse was thrilled when her "stick" resulted in a spurt of blood shooting onto the sheets. I almost fainted.

I was released to go home on the afternoon of the third day, after my oxygen level measured above 90 all day and I had demonstrated some clearing in my bronchial tubes. (I had also put on makeup to make me look healthier.)

Before my discharge, the hospital called my pharmacy with prescriptions for all the meds I was taking along with an albuterol nebulizer.

When I got home, I was feeling better, but tired — after spending the last three days in bed. Go figure.

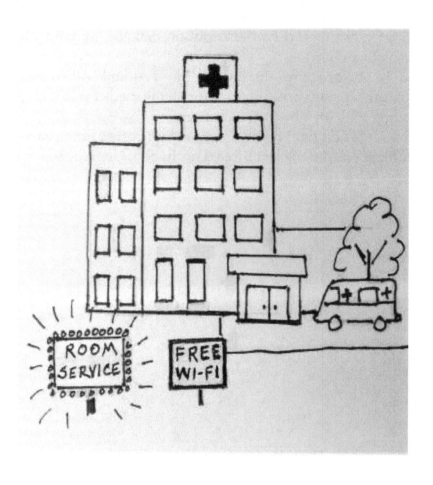

Chapter Twenty-two

Designing my Own Hospital

May 23 - 25, 2019

I spent the next couple of days at home recuperating. I was feeling much better, thanks to the excellent care I had received at the Fort Loudoun Medical Center. It appeared that the whole staff (volunteers, kitchen workers, CNAs, technicians, RNs, and the physicians) had lived up to the lofty goals for patient care that are set forth in the Patient's Medical Guidebook.

If anything was lacking, it was patient-friendly equipment and an ergonomically-designed space. Fort Loudoun is a modern hospital, built in 2004, and has the latest equipment. It's not like I had stayed in Bellevue Hospital in New York City where George Washington could have been treated. And I'm not singling out Fort Loudoun for awkward space design and unworkable equipment. Unfortunately, I've been in several hospitals over the years —in three over the last five months — to believe they're all the same.

Office design has evolved to make the workplace more comfortable and healthful, with desks that can be raised to standing height, ergonomic chairs, and non-glare lighting.

By contrast, hospital rooms are not designed for the comfort and well-being of the patient, but are booby-trapped with clumsy furniture and hard-to-use equipment. As I banged around my room for four days, I came up with some problem-solving ideas:

Tray tables.

Problem: They're too heavy for a weakened patient to move around. They have controls that are out of reach and a base that's wishbone-shaped that gets caught on the legs of the bed. (My table was fitted with useless plastic compartments at both ends that couldn't accommodate even a pair of glasses. The lower pull-out tray was locked on the side that faced me.)

Solution: Attach a light-weight hinged plastic tray to the side of the bed that can swing up and lock in place, and then drop down again when not needed.

IV stands.

Problem: They're top-heavy and unwieldy. Their bases have splayed legs that make them difficult to move them around other objects.

Solution: They could have round bases with hidden wheels underneath.

Beds.

Problem: The cables of the TV/call remote, phone, and additional bed control remotes slip down through the side rails to the floor and out of reach.

Solution: A caddie could be attached to the top of the rails to hold all of the controls for ready access.

Gowns.

Snaps and ties make it hard for the wearer to open and close the garment, particularly if they're in the back.

Solution: Replace snaps and ties with Velcro strips sewn on horizontally to allow for easy closing, opening, and adjusting for the size of the patient.

White Boards in the rooms.

Problem: They contain information for the patient's benefit but are too far away from the bed to be readable by most patients. They tend to be cluttered with too much data, such as the eight goals of the nursing staff that are included in the Patient Guide book. A graphic showing icon faces from smiling to cringing, representing pain from 0 to 10, lack definitions. Finally, there wasn't enough space to write the names of each day's nursing staff the patient needed to see.

Solution: White Boards should have a template designating space for necessary information to be written large enough to be read from across the room.

I know hospital rooms must house a lot of mechanical devices, but patients should be able to get out of bed without encountering obstacles. Getting out of bed, I had to twirl my IV stand around the legs of the bed, then shove the tray table and a heavy recliner out of the way. I could have called for a nurse, but I figured other patients were more in need.

I would also like to see a variety of room colors; and hallway colors that could identify locations.

I don't think there have been many improvements in the design of hospital rooms. The rooms I've been in lately are similar to my room when I had my tonsils out at the age of eight.

When the oversight nurse visited me to inquire about my stay before I checked out, I told her I received great care and then mentioned the design problems I saw along with my possible solutions. She said she'd raise the issues at the next Administrator's meeting.

I wish all administrators would stay overnight in their hospitals to experience what it's like to be a patient there. That might bring about some changes.

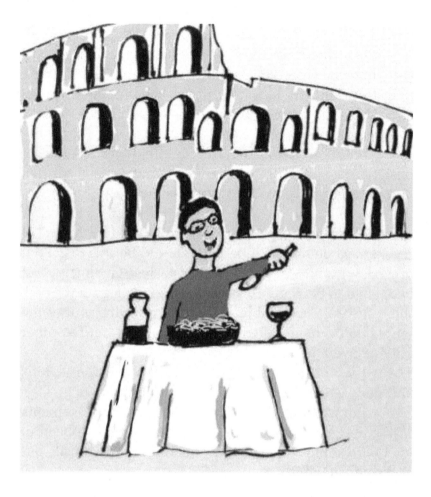

"This is fantastico! I'm in no hurry to get back home."

Chapter Twenty-three

Sure, Go on Vacation

May 28, 2019

I felt nervous checking into the cancer clinic for my last appointment in May since it was less than a week after being released from the hospital and I was still on medications for bronchitis. I was worried the staff wouldn't think I was healthy enough to take chemotherapy.

My first stop was the fusion room to have my blood drawn for lab analysis that would show my white blood cell count and other factors to determine my ability to tolerate treatment.

After the fusion room, Jim and I walked around to the doctor's waiting area. When I was called in, the nurse advised me that I wouldn't be seeing Dr. Feng today as he was on vacation in Italy. *What?!* I could only think he must have forgotten I had an appointment with him that day. The nurse said I would be seeing Ashley, the Nurse Navigator, who had my record and Dr. Feng's notes. Well...okay.

Next, I was asked to weigh in. Standing on the scale, I was shocked to see that I had lost seven pounds in the last two weeks. Normally, I would have been pleased with a weight loss, but I had been on prednisone since I was last here, which had increased my appetite. I knew I had been eating more, not less, so it was worrisome that I had lost weight.

A nurse showed us to an examining room where she took my vitals, which were good. Ashley soon came in with my lab results. Surprisingly, all my counts were normal for the first time. My white blood cell count was even down, although I still had bronchitis. Ashley was more pleased to see that I wasn't swollen from the extra-strength doses of steroids I've taken over the past two weeks.

She cautioned me to not be too concerned about my weight loss as it could be due to many factors that weren't problematic, including being in the hospital for four days. That seemed reasonable although I had eaten full meals and desserts during my stay.

We went over my physical condition during the past two weeks, including the skin rashes, my hospitalization for bronchitis, and my mammogram that showed the shrunken tumor.

As we talked about the mammogram, I asked if the number of my chemo treatments could now be reduced, since the tumor was almost non-existent after three cycles, or six sessions.

Ashley referred to her notes. "No, it looks like Dr. Feng wants you on a safe course of six-cycles. He might reduce the number with this report," she agreed. "You can talk to him about that after he comes back from vacation."

My mind conjured up an image of him relaxing on some palazzo sipping wine and tucking into a plate of pasta, in no rush to get back to decrease the number of my cycles of chemotherapy.

On our way out the door, Ashley offered some consolation. "Dr. Feng might lower the dosage of Abraxane or Neulasta if your rash comes back before next week." Swell.

Walking into the chemo room to the far end, I saw the place was nearly deserted, probably due to the Memorial Day holiday.

As we sat down near the snack table, I noticed there were no other women in the area; only a few elderly men who were either sleeping or resting. It was very quiet.

For a special treat that day there were homemade raspberry cookies we sampled with a cup of coffee.

The chemo session went without incident and was well-timed as I had just finished reading and sending emails when my bell dinged.

I was off for another week, hoping I wouldn't break out in rashes. My pharmacy had a back-up prescription for prednisone, just in case.

Hopefully, Dr. Feng will have finished touring Italy and be back at work to help me out.

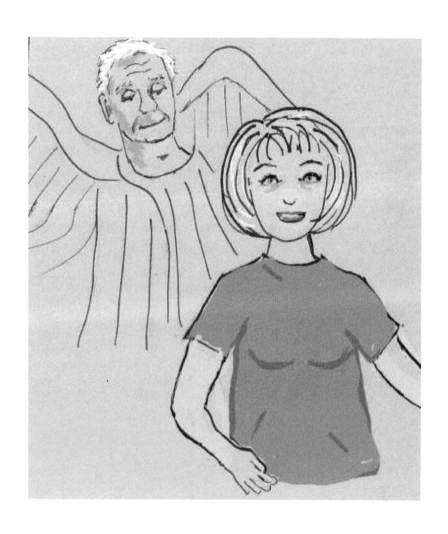

"Do I hear bells? I think I do!"

Chapter Twenty-four

An Angel on my Shoulder

June 4, 2019

The first Tuesday in June turned out to be my best day at the Tennessee Cancer Specialists clinic, although it didn't start out well. I had been moving like a sloth all morning, my gums hurt, and my skin was tingling with another emerging rash.

I was also feeling stressed about talking to Dr. Feng about decreasing my chemo treatments, fearing he would be adamant that I complete all six cycles. After four cycles I was miserable with additional side effects like lethargy, aching joints, mouth thrush, and skin rashes. I just wanted to be done with treatments to start feeling better again.

Walking through the double doors, I pulled back my shoulders and forced a smile for the receptionist. It wasn't her fault I felt so lousy. She greeted me warmly and handed me the form to fill out to note any new symptoms, meds, or procedures since the last visit. Jim and I were directed to wait near the laboratory.

Sitting down, I took the pen and started stabbing the boxes with check marks. Fatigue — check, shortness of breath — check, change in taste of food — check -- weight loss — check — depression — check. In my mood I considered putting a mark by vision problems, but I'd been farsighted for years.

After the blood drawing, Jim and I headed to the doctor's area where I had my vitals taken and was weighed. I was relieved that I had put back two pounds, to be reassured that I wasn't "wasting away." (I'm actually in no danger of that.)

In the examining room, we waited more than twenty minutes until Dr. Feng tapped on the door and strode in, smiling and extending his hand. I asked him how his vacation was. He said he had enjoyed Italy with his family but was glad to be home. I was glad he was home, too.

He sat down by the computer and pulled up my records. As he read the recent tests and lab results, I asked him if he would consider shortening my chemo treatments since I had gotten a "clean" mammogram. To my surprise, he nodded in agreement.

"I think today we finish up," he said.

I stared at him, open-mouthed.

"I'd have to argue with Humana for more fusions after what mammogram showed," he conceded.

I took a deep breath to take in the good news. Wow. I felt my mood elevate at this turning point in my cancer treatment.

Dr. Feng assured me there were still safeguards in place; that I would need to have a CT scan that would be more definitive than the mammogram. Then I'd have the surgery to remove any affected tissue, followed by weeks of radiation, and finishing up with a final scan. It was still a pretty long road, but the worst of it was over. I wouldn't feel sick and be in pain every day.

In the fusion room, I felt new energy and a return of optimism. I told every nurse that came near me that this was my last day.

"We'll have to ring the bells for you," they each said. I felt a warm glow. I couldn't wait for the celebration. Unfortunately, my treatment was delayed by the preparation of the Abraxane that was taking longer than usual.

When the bag was brought over and hung on the IV stand, I sneered up at it. *This is your last shot at me. Let's see what you've got!*

The extra time it took to prepare hadn't been a problem as I was enjoying my conversation with an attractive lady in the next chair. Peggy wasn't there for cancer treatments. She had had colon cancer forty years ago, but came once a month for hemoglobin infusions to build up her resistance to infection. She said with the infusions, she hadn't been sick a day for the last two years; that she was doing pretty well for being ninety. I couldn't believe she was that old. She still lived in her own home, and drove when necessary. Her daughter would be picking her up that day.

Peggy had inspired me with her spirit and her healthy looks. I told her that it was my last day there for chemotherapy but that I had enjoyed meeting and talking with her. She congratulated me for coming through a hard time.

As my bottle of Abraxane dripped out, I noticed that all the nurses were busy attending other patients. One finally broke free to unhook me and tape the last Neulasta patch on my arm. When she didn't say anything about it being my last day, I realized they had all forgotten and wouldn't be ringing the bells for me. I tried to shrug it off. I had gotten a great send-off from Peggy.

When I walked out of the fusion room for the last time, I imagined I had an angel on my shoulder ringing a bell. Maybe it was Clarence from "It's a Wonderful Life," finally getting his wings to help me on my way.

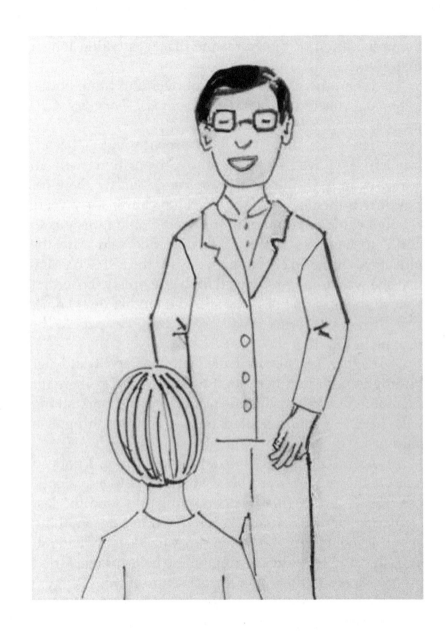

"I got the results back from all your scans and your MRI, Mrs. Peyton. You're not claustrophobic."

Chapter Twenty-five

Life After the Chemo Club

June 11 – 19, 2019

A week after my last treatment in the Tuesday Chemo Club I expected all my side effects to ease, but that was not the case. One night I felt itchy behind my knees and discovered clusters of red bumps. That wasn't even listed in my cancer notebook. I thought maybe I should report it to the clinic as a newly-discovered drug reaction. Or not. I also had swollen fingers I had never seen listed. And I barely had enough breath to walk up my driveway to the mailbox. I may have just been an oddity.

Penciling in eyebrows one morning to give my face some expression, I wondered how long it would take for real hair growth. I thought it would probably be several months until I could go without a wig. I kept it in a cabinet near the front door for when I went out. Indoors I avoided catching my reflection in the mirrors.

To stimulate my appetite, I had started making recipes from cookbooks, like lasagna that had enough seasoning to stimulate my appetite. I froze most of it so I'd have easy dinners later on.

On June 12, I had to report to Parkwest for a CT scan of my abdomen, as Dr. Feng had ordered as a "safeguard" before having my lumpectomy.

On that Friday, I had an appointment at a urologist's office for an ultrasound for my lower GI area that Dr. Feng had also ordered.

On that Saturday Jim and I drove up to Parkwest for my MRI, the last scan I'd have before surgery. My appointment was for 4:00; later than I had ever been scheduled at the hospital. When we arrived at 3:45, we were the only people in the lobby and as far as we could see into other areas.

We checked in with an intake worker at the desk in the empty out-patient waiting room, and a radiology nurse immediately appeared to escort me back to the MRI area. I figured she was probably anxious to finish her work day to go home.

After I changed into a short-sleeved robe, she came to my room and led me back to the chilly radiology room. Helping me onto the table, she instructed me to lie flat on my stomach.

"Are you comfortable?" she asked. Who wouldn't be comfortable wearing a flimsy nightgown in a cold room, lying face down on a board? When I complained that a table edge was digging into my sternum, she found a pad to put under me that made it much better. She then stretched me out in both directions and warned me not to move. Retreating to the safety of the back of the machine, she called out, "Here we go!" in an excited voice like it was a ride in an amusement park.

For the next half an hour I was subjected to the same ear-shattering buzzing, knocking, and whirring sounds I had endured once before.

Then it was over and all was quiet. Moments later I was helped off the table.

The next Tuesday Jim and I went to the cancer clinic to be advised of the results of all the scans. If none showed tumor activity, that would support the current plan of discontinuing chemo treatments. I didn't want to think about the alternative.

After I had my blood drawn, we walked over to the doctor's area where I was called into an examining room to see Dr. Feng. After a few suspenseful minutes, he knocked, simultaneously opening the door. Reaching out to shake my hand, he grinned and said he had "pretty good" news. *Just "pretty good?"* I held my breath.

Settling himself on a stool behind the computer, he brought up a screen with my appointments, treatments, and tests. He said he was looking at the CT of my chest, abdomen and pelvis. "Do you have a lung doctor?" he asked. *Lung doctor?* "Pulmonary doctor," he clarified.

"No, why?"

"You have COPD and pneumonia. What antibiotic did you get in the hospital?" Since I didn't have a ready answer, he pulled up the relevant record. "Doxycycline. That's good." *Apparently not good enough*, I thought glumly.

The "good news" was that there were no tumors on any of the scans so I would proceed to surgery in a couple weeks or so.

When we checked with the schedulers before we left, I was given a pre-op appointment with Dr Gibson for June 24. I had last seen him back in January when he inserted my port. A pulmonary doctor's office would be calling me to set up an appointment.

I left with a diagnosis of COPD and pneumonia, but I was (nearly) cancer-free so I felt I was in "pretty good" shape.

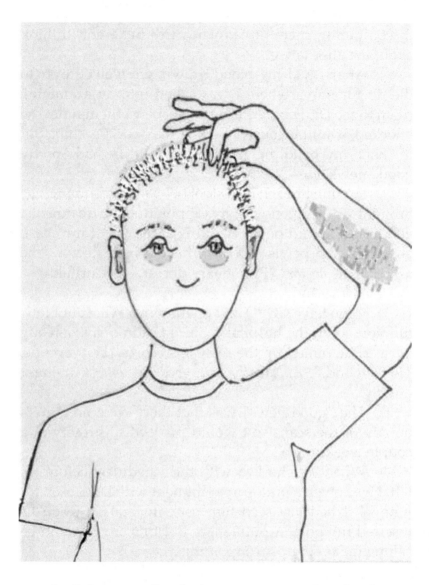

And they say that hair grows even after death.

Chapter Twenty-six

Planning for Surgery

June 30 – July 16, 2019

On the last day of June, Jim and I met with Dr. Gibson to discuss my case and to schedule what he termed my "wire-guided partial mastectomy, right axillary sentinel nod biopsy, adjacent tissue transfer and portacath removal." Easy for him to say.

Unfortunately, the first date that was available for surgery was July 30. According to Dr. Gibson, I needed at least four to six weeks to recover from chemotherapy, which was concluded on June 4th, and he needed to find an opening in his surgery schedule. I was always reminded how many cancer patients there were.

I was still experiencing side effects from chemotherapy so I knew that I wasn't ready to undergo surgery for a while, anyway. My chemo rash had returned, appearing where I didn't know I had places. Besides that, most days I had little energy, bordering on stupor, and I still had little appetite. Nothing tasted very good.

On the positive side, I was sporting "peach fuzz" on my head. I had been concerned I might not regrow hair as some people who have had multiple cancers and chemotherapy treatments never do. I was months away from having hair I would need to brush, but at least my scalp was covered.

After meeting with Dr. Gibson, we left his office in Parkwest Tower with a sheaf of papers of surgical instructions, new medications, and ancillary appointments. I only hoped he would remember my case when I'd see him a month later.

In the meantime, I was busy with painting projects around the house to keep up my spirits. The day before I had painted the garage floor to cover spatter that looked like a crime scene. Now that it was spotless, I hated to even drive the car over it.

* * *

By mid-July I still associated Tuesday with Chemo Club, although my last session had been six weeks earlier. I was then using Tuesday as a marker to evaluate any progress back to normalcy. When I walked the dog, I found that I could go a block further than the week before, and could climb a third hill. My rash had subsided to mostly tiny scabs left from scratching. In general, I had more energy. I no longer flopped on the couch in the afternoon, unable to move for an hour. Mentally, I felt more positive, looking ahead to my future.

Then, there was my hair. Or lack of. Pale blonde fuzz had sprouted but it was still less than two inches long. Every morning, the first thing I did was to grab hairs on the top of my head to see if they had grown any overnight; but I could never see any difference.

There was by then a shadow where my eyebrows had been that made penciling more accurate. I could feel emerging eyelashes with my fingertips, although none were visible or capable of holding mascara. At least I could use makeup on the rest of my face to give me some color and definition. I still wore my wig to cover my (nearly) bald head anytime I would leave the house, although I had gotten to the point where I wore a head scarf when I worked in the backyard; but not in the front yard. Inside the house, I continued to take off my wig, but kept it handy. I shampooed it every other day to keep it fresh.

I loved it when I was out and strangers would compliment me on "my hair." I never corrected them. It was my hair. I had bought it.

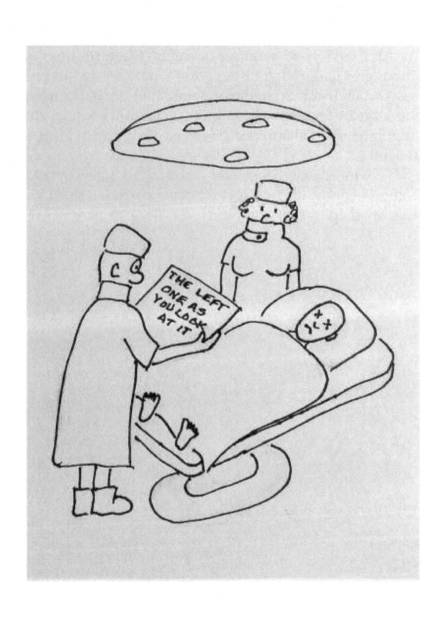

Chapter Twenty-seven

Surgery

July 23-30, 2019

A week before my surgery Jim and I drove to Parkwest for my "Pre-Admission testing." I wondered how they would "test" me for surgery.

Our first stop was registration. We had only just sat down in the waiting area when my pager buzzed and an Intake worker appeared to take us back to her office. After the usual preliminary questions, I was given a ream of paper to sign. In looking over the Patient's Rights and Responsibilities, I noted there were several areas of patient complaints that the hospital would help you file. Really? I saw that one has the right to designate any person as a visitor, or deny any would-be visitor. The statement concerning the patient's responsibility was "to communicate and cooperate with the medical staff, safeguard your valuables, and meet your financial obligations." Seemed fair.

At the end of the interview we walked over to the inpatient waiting area where I was quickly called. That interview covered previous surgeries and current medications. A knock at the door announced an anesthetic nurse who entered and asked a few questions about my surgery, like "which side is Dr. Gibson operating on?" *They didn't know?* And, what was my experience with anesthesia. I wondered what they did with people who couldn't tolerate anesthesia — give them whiskey and a washcloth to bite down on?

Finally, the Intake worker rattled off the list of pre-surgery instructions, all of which were expected, like — you must have someone drive you home after your operation, and no eating after midnight. *Who eats after midnight?* But there was one true hardship: no makeup. Are you kidding? I wasn't worried about the surgery, but not being allowed to wear makeup was going too far. I could only hope Dr. Gibson recognized me to perform the right surgery. Without having hair or any makeup on, he might think I was his appendectomy.

Tuesday, July 30, 2019.

I stayed overnight in our townhouse as I did before all my appointments when Jim would accompany me. We planned to leave early in the morning.

The radio sprang to life at 6:15 a.m., but I didn't. After a couple minutes, I forced myself to get up and I lumbered into the bathroom. Following doctor's instructions, I showered with Dial anti-bacterial soap. After toweling off, I examined the sprigs of hair on my head in the mirror, looking for growth, and winced at the sight of my pale face I wasn't allowed to bring to life with any makeup. I had to remind myself to appreciate this time of day as I'd feel and look a lot worse later on.

We hit the road by 7:15 a.m. and arrived at our first stop, the Comprehensive Breast Center, down the street from Parkwest, right at 8:00. I was the first patient of the day.

The initial task was to have a mammogram. I guess I can't have too many of them. This would be my fourth in seven months.

After that, I returned to my examining room. A nurse came in and advised me that she would be inserting a wire into my areole where Dr. Gibson would make his incision. Egads. She first injected my breast with a numbing solution, which hurt before it did any numbing. After she put the wire in, I couldn't even look at it.

I wondered how I would get to the hospital. In the waiting room, the nurse informed Jim that she would take me by wheelchair through a corridor that now connected Physicians Plaza, where we were, with the main hospital building

Jim left to leave the car with the hospital valet service. We met up with him in the crowded waiting room for outpatients where I would wait to have X-rays taken for a current picture to aid my surgeon.

After that, Jim and I went on to the surgery waiting room that was also nearly filled. The woman behind the desk explained the tracking system to us so Jim could follow my progress by locating my number on a chart.

From the waiting room, we followed an aide to my assigned pre-surgery room — another chilly room, sparsely furnished with a bed and a couple chairs.

I changed into the gown that was left for me and slid between the cold sheets. Fortunately, a nurse soon arrived with an air-filled warming blanket for me and a cotton blanket for Jim.

She informed us that Dr. Gibson was just starting the surgery before mine, so it would be over an hour before he would be coming in to talk to us about my procedure.

It was 11:30 a.m. The anesthetist came in and answered some of our questions about the timing of the whole process. He estimated that I would be going into surgery about 1:00, then on to recovery between 2:00 and 2:30 where I'd remain until 3:30 to 4:00. We decided this was a good time for Jim to go home, take of the dog, and to come back by 3:00.

Sometime after he left, a female aide and a male orderly came in. Pulling up my side rails, they tucked the blanket around me and rolled my bed out of the room and down the hallway to the operating room.

I was feeling a little nervous but excited to get the surgery over with — and to have that wire removed. It made me wince every time I caught sight of it.

As I was wheeled into the all-white room, I noticed three other young aides in scrubs cleaning and organizing instruments and clearing tables. They were all moving to the beat of Carly Simon's hit song from the '70s, "You're so Vain" playing on a radio. I figured I was the only one there who had heard that the lyrics referred to Warren Beatty. They had probably never heard of Warren Beatty.

A surgical nurse introduced herself just before she clamped an oxygen mask over my face. At least, she said it was oxygen. I felt myself getting woozy, which is the last thing I remember before I woke up in recovery being attended to by another nurse.

My first sensation was the discomfort caused by layers of ace bandaging wrapped around my torso from under my arms down to my waist. It reminded me of when Scarlet O'Hara's Mammy tied her into a corset as she hung onto the bedpost.

Dr. Gibson came in to see how I was doing and cautioned me to leave the bandaging on for forty-eight hours —two whole days. He said it was important to "hold things together" while I healed. I could take it off any time on the third day. He also advised me to keep pressure off the incision under my arm where my sentinel lymph node had been removed.

When I went to bed that night, I lay flat on my back, barely able to breathe with the bandaging digging into my chest, and holding my right arm up above my head, hitting the headboard. (Don't tell Dr. Gibson, but I loosened the bandaging a little so I could get some sleep.)

I then had only two days to get myself together enough to look and act somewhat normal for a planned trip to Chicago to visit with family. Good thing I wouldn't be doing a lot of sightseeing.

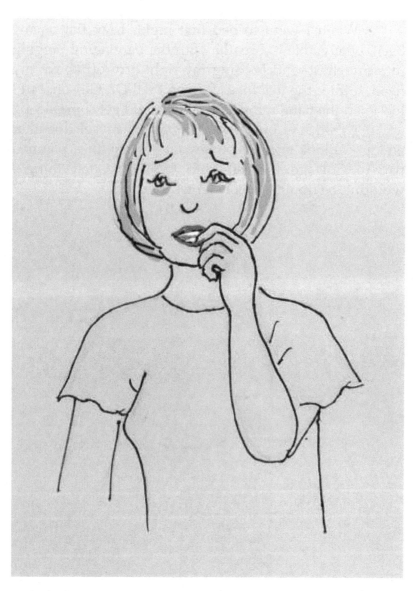

"It could be good news, but what if it's bad news? Of course, I could call and find out."

Chapter Twenty-eight

A Turning Point

August 6, 2019

After a good weekend with family, we returned from Chicago about nine o'clock Monday evening.

Walking into the darkened kitchen, the answering machine was blinking "2." Jim hit the Play button for the first message. The automated voice informed us the message was recorded on Friday, August 2. "This is for Cheryl Peyton," an unfamiliar female voice said, and then went on. "This is Vanessa, Dr. Gibson's nurse. I'm calling to see how you're doing after your surgery on Tuesday. "

I thought, okay, fine. I would call her back in the morning to let her know I was doing well.

Jim pressed the button for the second message that was recorded on Sunday at 6:30 p.m. "Hi, Cheryl. This is Vanessa again, from Dr. Gibson's office. Please call me back at your earliest convenience. I have the results of your pathology from your surgery I'd like to give you. Again, my number again is . . ."

Why would she call me on a Sunday evening from home to give me my biopsy results and request that I call her back ASAP? At this point, my "earliest convenience" was the next morning.

The next day I woke up with a start, my thoughts focused on the call I would make to Vanessa. Should I phone her as soon as I got dressed? No. it was too early. I'd take the dog out first.

After I came back in, I stared at the silent phone. Should I call now? No, I'd have breakfast first. If Vanessa had called with bad news, I wouldn't be able to eat after hearing it.

I opened the newspaper to distract me while I ate my muffin with tomato juice, and coffee. I found I couldn't absorb what I was reading, so I put the paper down. My mind wouldn't rest until I called the nurse.

Having finished my breakfast, I walked over to the counter, picked up the phone, took a deep breath, and punched in the number that Vanessa had left. It turned out to be the surgical group. I told the receptionist I was answering Vanessa's call. I was quickly transferred and Vanessa came on the line. I explained why I hadn't been able to call sooner. "Oh, that's fine. I just wanted to let you know that the biopsies on the breast tissue and the lymph node were all clear."

I couldn't believe it. Clear. This was the first time since early January that I knew the cancerous tumor was totally gone, leaving no cells behind. I couldn't help but sound a little weepy as I thanked her for the report. She understood. "I wanted to give you the good news as soon as I could. I'm so happy for you."

She couldn't have been as happy as I was. I knew I would still need radiation treatments, but I'd enjoy the break until then — and every breakfast for some time to come.

* * *

The following week I had a follow-up appointment with Dr. Gibson. After examining me, he pronounced the surgery a success and that the site was healing nicely.

I still had to be protective of the area as the incision and the former site of the port were still tender. What was remarkable was that I didn't have any noticeable scar or depression in my breast.

The next subject we discussed was radiation. Dr. Gibson felt I should have a total of thirty treatments given over six weeks, five days a week. He had referred me to Dr. Joseph Meyer, a radiation oncologist, at East Tennessee Radiation Oncology Clinic, to make the final decision.

Dr. Gibson said I'd be hearing from Dr. Meyer's office to schedule an appointment for three weeks in the future. The clinic was affiliated with Parkwest and located near the hospital in the Thompson Cancer Survival Center.

I thought that sounded like a good place to go for my last cancer treatments.

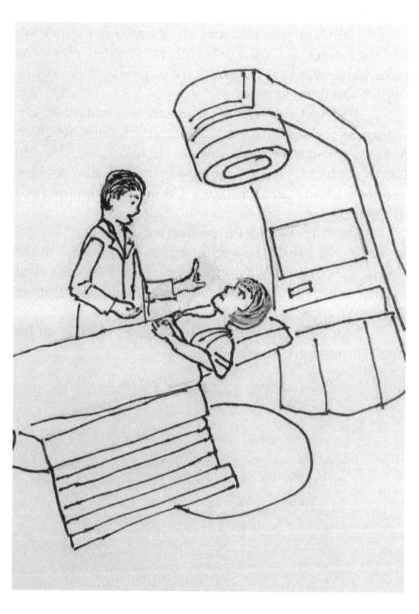

"Hold on, Mrs. Peyton. I have to tell George I won this time with three x's on the diagonal."

Chapter Twenty-nine

"X" Marks the Spot

August, 2019 - September 20, 2019

In the month following my surgery, I was re-examined by both Dr. Gibson and Dr. Feng, and had several scans performed by radiologists; all of whom reached the same conclusion — no cancer had been detected and my anatomy was reasonably returned to its pre-cancerous condition.

My hair was thickening some, but was growing slowly, not yet over two inches long. I had started noticing women whose hair was styled in cuts as short as my hair. I briefly considered going bare-headed and rocking the look with large hoop earrings, bright lipstick, and abstract prints, but then realized I was more comfortable with my regular chin-length style, even though the look was then contrived with a wig.

I was scheduled to begin my five-day-a-week radiation treatments on September 23 and they were expected to continue for six weeks. In the first three weeks of September, I had been to the radiation clinic three times for consultation, X-rays, and examinations, concluding with a "marking session" when technicians drew x's on my breast with a Magic Marker to pinpoint where they should aim the radiation. My chest looked like a map of a military operation.

On the Friday before I started my daily treatments, I had an appointment at the clinic for a "dry run." I had been cautioned to always be on time for my treatments as the clinic runs a tight schedule to get patients in and out of the two radiation rooms. I had been promptly seen on my three visits.

So, I was surprised when I arrived at 12:50 for my 1:00 appointment to find fourteen people in the waiting room (including some spouses, I assumed). In the first fifteen minutes, only one person had been called, followed by intervals of several minutes between patients being called for treatment.

After I had been there for forty minutes with people who were there when I walked in, I went over to the desk to ask if there was a reason for the delay. The receptionist apologized and said that the computers had been down all morning in the hospital and the satellite clinics. Only two radiology patients had been treated there before the crash, so the other morning patients were given afternoon times, doubling up the schedule. I was glad to know the wait was due to some unusual technical problem, but it would have been better to have been told when we arrived.

When I resumed my seat, I shared the information with the others sitting nearby. Several of the patients voiced relief in having an explanation, saying they had never seen the waiting room so crowded. One woman said she recognized patients still waiting who usually were leaving when she arrived.

This discussion opened up more conversation about treatment. I shared that this was my first time for radiation. The woman on my left said that this was her 28th treatment. Pulling her blouse open, she showed us her red, blistered upper chest she said was a third-degree burn. I had only seen that serious a burn in pictures of people who had survived a fire. She said she was grateful to have been given ointments and wrappings from one of the nurses that day.

On my right, a frail-looking bald woman, who had sat bent over since I had sat down, looked up with a wan smile. "This is my 29th treatment," she said in a raspy voice. "I have only one more to go."

Everyone mumbled congratulations and good wishes.

She turned to me and shook a bony finger. "Be sure to use salves so you don't get too burned. They've helped me."

A heavyset woman across from the three of us spoke up that she was missing out on a trip to Costco with her husband who had just left after waiting with her for over an hour.

The conversation continued for several minutes, sharing tips and experiences.

Finally, I was called in and escorted down the hallway to a large dimly-lit room where I was asked to undress down to the waist behind a portable changing screen and to slip on a paper gown.

After I lay down on the cot, the radiologist made a few more markings on me before operating the rotating heads. When I sat up, I saw that my chest looked like a game of tic tac toe with x's and o's. I asked the doctor if I needed to cover all of these marks with plastic when I showered.

He shook his head. "No, that's not necessary. We'll probably need to re-mark you during treatments as you lose or gain weight."

I thought, what am I in for? I might change shape enough to move x's and o's around on my chest? And would I be burned to a crisp in the process?

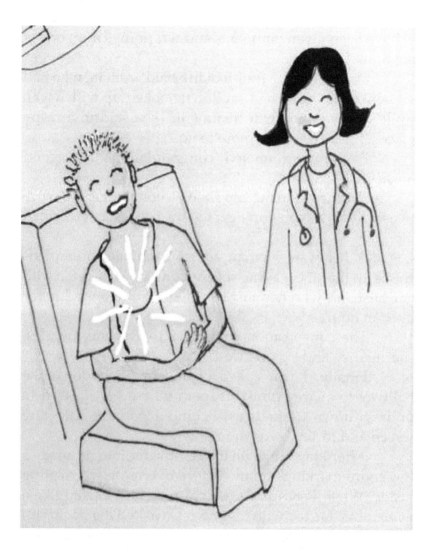

"You look absolutely radiant, Mrs. Peyton!"

Chapter Thirty

Becoming Radiant

October, 2019

By the second week in October I had been to the radiology clinic ten times — one third of the way through my course of treatment. My skin had become dry and papery, even with the salves, but, thankfully, it wasn't irritated or burned. My weight was stable, so I assumed my markings were still good.

I had enough energy to work even more on the house as I planned to put it on the market in a month. I looked forward to resuming my married life with Jim in our townhouse.

I still had more painting to do even though I had gone through at least thirty gallons at last count, including indoor and outdoor paint and concrete stain. It had taken me most of the summer to paint faux bricks on the driveway. I still had to finish smaller projects both inside and outside. I had just painted the heat pump on the side of the house to cover the rusty fan cover and the weathered sides so it wouldn't attract negative attention from a would-be buyer.

By the third week of daily appointments at the radiation clinics, I was on automatic pilot: I would leave the house at precisely 1:30 to arrive at exactly 2:10, to be called in at 2:15 on the dot.

Since the same people came at the same time every day, the place had a familiar and friendly vibe. Like the bar in the sit-com "Cheers," everybody knew your name and seemed happy to see you. The atmosphere was laid-back and relaxed.

I remember one day, when a nurse came out to the waiting room to get me to go back for treatment, she mentioned that the lady ahead of me was just getting dressed so we should take our time. In unison, we started walking in exaggerated slow motion down the long hall, laughing at our silliness.

Another day, I sat next to a pleasant-looking woman in the waiting room I hadn't seen before. To make conversation, I asked the typical radiation-clinic question: "How many times do you have left?"

She shrugged and rolled her eyes. "I don't know. I just keep showing up. I figure when I've come enough times, they'll tell me to stay home."

I thought that said it all. We all came every day until we've absorbed our quota of rays and then we're released. It would be another month for me. I could be roasted before the turkey; and maybe I'd be wearing my own hair for Christmas. Cheers.

October 29, 2019

I had scheduled an appointment with an orthopedic surgeon to have my left ring finger straightened during the last week of my radiation treatment. The finger had been bending down for a couple of years due to a condition called Dupuytren's contracture.

At the beginning of the week I was still waiting to hear from Humana whether they would cover the expense of the treatment: a single injection of Xiaflex that cost $5,000.00. I had been advised it could take a couple weeks for the Board to research my request and make a decision. I wondered what questions they asked in their deliberations: "How much does this Cheryl use her left hand, anyway? Isn't she right-handed? And retired? Besides, she's got three other fingers and a thumb. What's the problem with one bent finger?"

Finally, on Monday, I received notice that the treatment had been approved. After all my medical expenses during the year I figured Humana probably had posted my picture on a dart board in their lunchroom.

One interesting fact about Dupuytren's contracture is that it's more common for people of northern European descent. I'm Swedish on both sides going back generations, so I had those darn Vikings to thank for that finger.

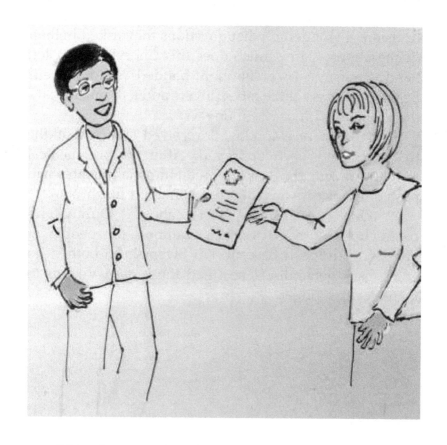

"Here's your clean bill of health, Mrs. Peyton. Hopefully, we won't be seeing much more of you."

Chapter Thirty-one

All Good (and Bad) Things Must Come to an End

November through December, 2019

On November 6th I drove out of the parking lot of the East Tennessee Oncology Radiation Clinic after my last radiation session. It had been number thirty-five.

I had finally completed all my cancer treatments — chemotherapy, surgery, and radiation — after ten months. I started on the process January 11, 2019, having my first mammogram that pictured the tumor I had felt two weeks before Christmas.

After that, I had been put through a battery of tests to confirm the location, size, and cellular composition of the tumor including: diagnostic mammograms, ultrasounds, MRIs and CT scans.

In all of my visits to Parkwest and their satellite cancer centers, I had always been treated with compassion, kindness, and expert care and had a laugh or two along the way.

As I drove away from the radiation clinic, I thought how much I had enjoyed the daily joshing with the radiologists and nurses. As I left, I told them I'd miss stopping by every afternoon to strip for them and they advised me not to flash people at Walmart's. Fair enough.

I knew I would be having more tests and scans to check for a recurrence of the disease, but I left the radiation clinic that day feeling confident that I had conquered cancer for the time being and I had been given a certificate from the Radiation Clinic to prove it. It read, "Congratulations, you did it."

When I returned home, I picked up a message from my realtor that my house had been selected by HGTV for an episode of House Hunters. I was elated that I had improved the property enough from being the neighborhood eyesore to being the "move-in-ready option" for home buyers on a national TV home design show.

December 23, 2019.

On the day before Christmas Eve I had to return to Ft. Loudoun hospital for more tests. My blood analysis at the cancer center two weeks earlier had revealed a spike in the tumor marker that led to speculation the cancer had returned and spread, possibly to my bones.

My morning began with an infusion of nuclear medicine that would have to course through me for several hours. Not to waste time while we waited, I was given a bone density test that proved to be brief and painless. I didn't know at the time I was being lulled into a false sense of security.

The next three hours, while I sat around to wait for the nuclear medicine to make its rounds, I was allowed to eat just a few crackers and encouraged to drink water.

When the time was up, a nurse came to get me for my scan. Lying on a narrow table, she bound my hands and feet and cautioned me not to move during the scan that would last an hour. By the time the scan was completed, my limbs had become numb.

Sitting up, I checked my watch. It was 3:30. It seemed like I should be able to go home, but I wasn't through yet.

As I waited in a lounge area, my nurse, Jennifer, brought me two large bottles of barium; one to drink to the bottom and the other to drink down to a black line near the bottom. "Don't drink past the line on the second bottle," Jennifer cautioned. Like I would try to get away with drinking more barium.

I needed all my will power as it was to get down the thick, white alkaline liquid. Then I had to wait an hour while it circulated. Finally, I had a CT scan. Stretching out on the cot to be slowly moved in and out of the machine seemed like a treat after drinking the barium.

I was finally released from the hospital at five o'clock. I had been there as long as some of the staff. Taking a deep breath, I pushed the door open and started toward my car that sat in the now nearly-deserted lot. Driving home, my thoughts turned to how I would be celebrating Christmas over the next two days.

Tennessee Cancer Specialists contacted me a few days later to inform me that all my scans were negative. I wasn't surprised.

Epilogue

I'm not an expert on cancer but I've learned a few things by being its victim three times. I've learned it doesn't have to be a death sentence. I've learned that there are improved diagnostic tests and more effective drugs being developed all the time to battle the disease. I've learned that there are caring, competent doctors and nurses who have devoted their careers to helping people survive its ravages. I've learned it helps to stay busy, focused, and to keep a positive attitude even when you're in pain. I've learned that cancer doesn't have to define you as a patient — you can be an active person, capable of growing and accomplishing new goals. I've learned that cancer can give you more appreciation of what's important in your life and not to worry about trivialities. Finally, I've learned who really cares about me and is always there to support me.

    I know that sometimes I was "wigged out" during the twelve months of tests and treatments. At times I succumbed to my fears, or became depressed by nagging pain or lack of energy, but more often I was hopeful and pushed myself to stay busy and productive.

    Toward the end of my treatment I had a DNA blood test that revealed I have inherited the gene mutation marker for cancer. I've traced it back to my father's mother, Annette, who died in 1940 at age 56 of ovarian cancer. Her daughter, my aunt, contracted breast cancer in her early thirties, but lived well into her eighties. Her daughter, my cousin, survived three bouts of breast cancer she was treated for several years ago.

There is no "cure" for cancer, but there are treatments that can eradicate it in the present.

I'm grateful for what cancer has taught me and that I've been restored to health thanks to my doctors, nurses, and technicians. I want to especially thank my husband who was always there for me; comforting me when I was down and celebrating with me when I rebounded.

I'm a lucky woman.

Made in the USA
Columbia, SC
13 July 2022